FOAM ROLLING

FOAM ROLLING

50 Exercises for Massage, Injury Prevention, and Core Strength

KARINA INKSTER, MA, PTS

Skyhorse Publishing

Skyhorse Publishing books may be purchased in bulk at special discounts for sales promotion, corporate gifts, fund-raising, or educational purposes. Special editions can also be created to specifications. For details, contact the Special Sales Department, Skyhorse Publishing, 307 West 36th Street, 11th Floor, New York, NY 10018 or info@skyhorsepublishing.com.

Skyhorse® and Skyhorse Publishing® are registered trademarks of Skyhorse Publishing, Inc.®, a Delaware corporation.

Visit our website at www.skyhorsepublishing.com.

10 9 8 7 6 5 4 3 2

Library of Congress Cataloging-in-Publication Data is available on file.

Cover design by Rain Saukas
Cover photo by John Watson of Image Maker Photographic Studio

ISBN: 978-1-63220-627-5
Ebook ISBN: 978-1-63220-761-6

Printed in China

CONTENTS

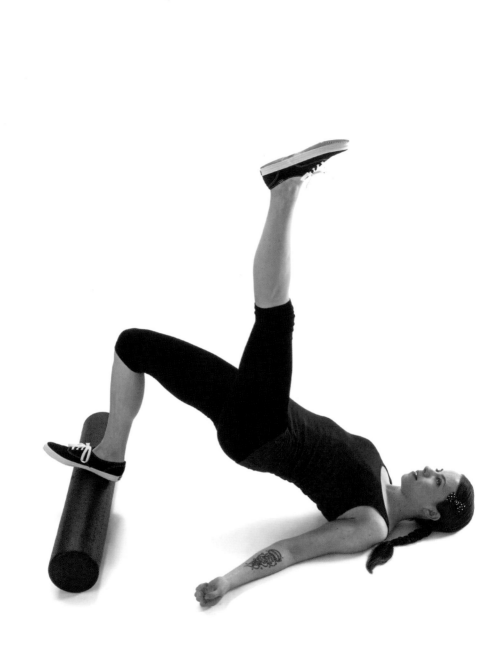

CHAPTER 1:
FOAM ROLLER BASICS

WHAT IS FOAM ROLLING AND HOW DOES IT WORK?

Foam rolling is a technique quickly making its way from physical therapists' offices into mainstream gyms, personal training studios, and homes everywhere. Foam rolling is most often used as a form of self massage, working out the soreness and tight spots in our muscles. It's much more economical than seeing a masseuse, athletic trainer, or other body-worker; plus, you're able to control precisely where to apply pressure, and how much.

A foam roller is a cylinder of dense foam, usually six inches in diameter. Typical lengths are one foot or three feet. You place the foam roller on the floor and use your own bodyweight to apply pressure to various muscle groups, slowly rolling back and forth across each muscle (e.g. upper back or hamstrings).

You may have heard many different terms being used to describe this practice, including "trigger point release" or "active release." You may have also heard the term "soft tissue mobilization," which is the physical therapy term for massage. The technical term for foam rolling, which I'll use in this book, is self-myofascial release, based on the word "fascia." And what is fascia, exactly? Let's take a look.

Foam rolling and its related physiological mechanisms are a relatively new area of research. Here's what we currently understand about fascia. Fascia is a dense layer in the human body that covers every structure, including muscles, organs, nerves, and blood vessels. It allows all our structures to function smoothly and slide without friction. When we overstress our muscles—due to overuse or perhaps an injury—the layers of fascia in our bodies can tear. Several layers of fascia can stick together when these tears don't heal properly. These are called adhesions. They can be painful, and they prevent our muscles from working properly. Self-myofascial release–putting pressure on adhesions–is thought to release adhesions, returning our muscles to optimal performance. Much like massage, foam rolling can help the muscles themselves to return to normal functioning if they're too tight, but much of the foam rolling benefit is thought to come from the action of fascia.

Much more research is needed to better undertand fascia and how foam rolling can affect it. For now, we can be fairly certain that foam rolling leads to neuromuscular relaxation. That means it can stimulate your brain to relax your muscles. While researchers get busy figuring out exactly what mechanisms are at play during foam rolling, let's focus on the fact that it feels great, eases tension in your muscles, and can potentially increase your mobility and accelerate your recovery after physical training.

WHAT IS FOAM ROLLING USED FOR?

Foam rolling is a way to release muscle tension and possibly even improve athletic performance.

Research studies are beginning to look into specific benefits of foam rolling, including–perhaps surprisingly–arterial function.[1] In one study, researchers investigated whether foam rolling particular muscle groups would affect arterial stiffness and vascular endothelial function. Endothelium is the inner lining of blood vessels. Participants were tested for brachial-ankle pulse wave velocity (a measure of arterial stiffness), blood pressure, heart rate, and plasma nitric oxide concentration (a measure of vascular endothelial function) after either foam rolling, or not foam rolling on separate days.

---

1   Okamoto, T., Masuhara, M., & Ikuta, K. (2014). Acute effects of self-myofascial release using a foam roller on arterial function. *Journal of Strength and Conditioning Research, 28*(1), p. 69-73.

Participants rolled the adductors (inner thigh muscles), hamstrings, quadriceps, iliotibial band (running along the outside of the thigh from the hip to the knee), and trapezius (an upper back muscle), self-adjusting the pressure applied to each muscle group by using their hands and feet to offset some of their bodyweight. After foam rolling, compared to the control trial, brachial-ankle pulse wave velocity significantly decreased, and plasma nitric oxide concentration significantly increased. This suggests that foam rolling can reduce arterial stiffness and improve vascular endothelial function.

Other benefits often associated with foam rolling are increased blood flow to muscles, injury prevention, increased flexibility, and reduced soreness after workouts. Many of these benefits need to be studied in greater depth by clinical researchers, but we can see from anecdotal evidence—and the rising popularity of foam rolling—that people who foam roll regularly experience some of these positive effects. Many of these benefits will be discussed in further detail in Chapter 2: Benefits of Foam Rolling.

Here are some thoughts from my fitness coach colleagues on using foam rollers with their clients (and on themselves), the benefits of regular foam rolling, and their "do's" and "don'ts."

Angela Kromidas (ACE Certification, PICP Level 3, Functional Movement Specialist) of You Wellness in Vancouver, BC uses foam rolling as a tool for recovery between her own athletic training sessions, as well as with her fitness coaching clients. Here's what she says about it.

The foam roller became a part of my world as a tool for my own recovery. Identifying the tight and/or sore spots and using the roller in those areas made a massive difference in my own growth and progress. Subsequently adding it to my training toolbox for my clients was a natural progression.

I now routinely use the foam roller with my clients, which has allowed them to see increased blood circulation. This aids in muscle recovery and leads to an overall increase in performance. Such a portable tool allows me to achieve greater participation from my clients. With a brief knowledge transfer, they are able to take the foam roller home and work with it on their own. This increased teamwork allows us to achieve enduring results, which leads to enhanced client loyalty.

Certified strength and conditioning specialist Faolan Dunphy of Speed Power Endurance Sport Performance, Conditioning, and Consulting shares with you his thoughts on the uses of foam rolling and the "do's" and "don'ts" he teaches his clients.

I allow my clients and athletes the choice to use foam rollers as an adjunct to their training programs; I include space in their written programs for them to include it, but I don't prescribe it as such. If they have time to include it as part of their soft tissue management and they find it beneficial, I will accept and encourage the psychological benefit even if there is limited supporting research for its physiological benefit at this time. I will also use it to treat myself when I can't get manual therapy. Reported benefits of foam rolling include decreased residual muscle tone or tightness, increased mobility and/or flexibility, and a general sense of ease.

Typically I suggest that the rolling be done to large masses of tissue, specifically the muscle bellies. Roll slowly yet fluidly to maintain or promote circulation and avoid over-compressing tissues and potentially causing contusions (bruising). Spend a little extra time on trigger points (particular "knotty" areas) to help decrease the tension within the fibers and the potential formation of nodules and/or adhesions.

Do get manual therapy (i.e. massage) to distract, or separate, fascial layers and adhesions, which foam rolling cannot do. Foam rolling is compressive in nature, whereas massage is distractive—therefore, rolling should not be used as a replacement for massage. Also, stretch using passive and active techniques to help prevent nodules and/or adhesions from forming in the first place, preferably immediately post-activity.

Stay away from rolling large connective tissues tracts (like the ilio-tibial band [IT band] or thoracolumbar fascia in the lower back area), as this can potentially cause greater adhesions to develop by mashing layers of connective tissue together, actually impeding the ability of muscle compartments to contract independently of other surrounding tissues. This essentially defeats the purpose of foam rolling.

Over the years I've used foam rollers and half rollers in a variety of different ways including as balance implements, for therapeutic or rehabilitative work, and even to beat up my clients a little when they get out of line (just kidding!).

ACE-certified personal trainer Gemma Doyle of Fierce Training, who has a post-graduate degree in sport and exercise science, gives recommendations for the best foam roller, and describes how she incorporates foam rolling into most sessions with her fitness coaching clients.

My roller of choice is *The GRID,* made by Trigger Point Performance. Although it's one of the pricier options, it is firmer than its foam counterparts and its longevity is second to none. It is, however, not for the faint hearted!

I believe that rolling and the use of a trigger point balls should be integral parts of every client's pre-workout routine. In my first session with new or prospective clients, I include a postural assessment and a comprehensive guide to foam rolling/trigger point release, and its benefits. I ask all my clients to arrive (as often as possible) at least 10 to 15 minutes early in order to roll correctly before their session begins.

The roller is extremely effective in preparing a client for safe movement and increased mobility, but it is temporary. If a client has mobility limitations and/or tissue adhesions the roller may not be enough to break down the fibrotic tissue.

Many people describe foam rolling as "fascia release," when a better way to educate our clients is to use the term "tissue release" because we are affecting more than just the fascia itself. I use foam rolling to prepare muscles for training, to re-hydrate damaged or tight tissues, and to improve mobility in a joint or extensibility in muscle tissue. I also like to use it as a tool to gauge the state of a client's body. When a client foam rolls before a workout, we can often detect overly tight areas or sore spots. We can then address these before training, thus avoiding injury.

When foam rolling, take your time and be gentle–you are not a pie crust! Don't rush. When you find a tender spot, stop and breathe. Make sure you cover all areas, especially the extra tight, nasty bits!

Certified Personal Trainer and Registered Fitness Leader Naomi Canales of Funky Fitness shares how she uses the foam roller with her clients, the benefits her clients see, and her top "do's" and "don'ts" of rolling.

Using a foam roller offers a number of benefits. As a myofascial release technique, it can be used to inhibit over-active muscles. I suggest to my clients to foam roll every second day to maximize its results. Foam rolling is especially helpful for some common ailments such as:

IT Band syndrome: to relax the hamstring and hip flexor while working on strengthening the glutes.

Tight glutes and calves: using your foam roller can help to relax tight or strained glutes and calves.

Runner's knee: pain at the front of the knee can be caused by tightness in the outside of the quad muscle, coupled with weakness on the inside quad. This causes a tracking problem with the kneecap. You can foam roll the outside of the quad to help it relax as you strengthen the inside.

Overall use of the foam roller can help to maintain muscle balance and prevent overuse, fatigue, and inactivity (which could lead to an injury). When injured it can help to deactivate overactive muscles so you can strengthen weak muscles. Work with a health and fitness professional to determine the exact cause of muscle imbalances, and what you should do to improve them.

Generally my clients enjoy having foam rolling as part of their programs, as it can promote feelings of relaxation. Plus, it just feels good–like a massage!

Often I train my clients to perform core work as they balance with their backs on a foam roller. This brings a whole new level to core stability training. One must get in touch with one's inner core muscles before attempting this. [Karina's note: see page 113 for core stability and strength exercises using the foam roller.]

Naomi's Do's and Don'ts:

Do roll slowly! Ten slow rolls in each position.

Don't roll over bones or joints!

Roll only when muscles are warm or after a workout.

If you find a painful area, hold that position until the area softens.

TYPES OF FOAM ROLLERS

The two most common types of foam rollers are circular and semicircular (often called "half rollers"). Circular rollers are usually six inches in diameter, and semicircular rollers are three inches in diameter. Both types come in lengths of either one foot or three feet. The exercises in this book use the longer rollers, since the one-foot rollers are too short to lie on lengthwise. Circular rollers are more unstable than semicircular rollers, which means they'll be more challenging to use, especially for core stability and strength exercises. If you're new to foam rolling, you may want to start with a semicircular roller and move to a circular one once you're comfortable with the "half" foam roller.

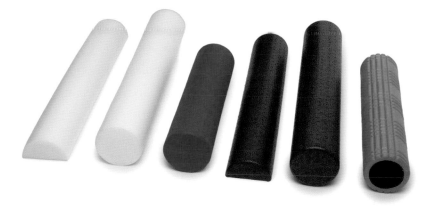

From left to right: low density (soft) half roller, low density full roller, medium density full roller, high density (hard) half roller, high density full roller, and The GRID roller (most intense for massage purposes).

Foam rollers come in a variety of densities. The harder, or more dense, the foam roller you use, the more "good pain" you're likely to feel. Softer foam rollers don't offer as much pressure on your soft tissue as do harder foam rollers. Unfortunately, there is no clinical research to date that tells us which type of roller is best. Most health and fitness professionals recommend starting with a softer foam roller—especially if your muscles are chronically tight and/or you have a sedentary job—and progressing to more dense versions as your muscles get accustomed to foam rolling.

Once you're comfortable with basic foam rolling and you experience minimal "good pain" in your muscles, you could consider the most intense foam roller of all: The GRID. Made by Trigger Point Performance, The GRID is a hollow tube of sturdy plastic covered with dense foam. Rather than being smooth like other foam rollers, The GRID is covered in ridges with areas of differing densities for a more intensive massage. It's much more durable than standard foam rollers, and even though it's hollow, it can support up to 500 pounds. It's five inches in diameter instead of the usual six. Most commonly found in the 13-inch length, it's also available in a 26-inch length. Because it's lightweight and hollow, the 13-inch *GRID* is a great travel option.

CHAPTER 2:
BENEFITS OF FOAM ROLLING

Foam rolling has many benefits, but if you're working on correcting a specific problem (like loosening tight hip flexors, increasing mobility in the upper back, fixing a lower back problem, etc.), there may be modalities that work better for your issue than foam rolling. Make sure you see a qualified professional to see what would work best for your specific situation. For overall mobility, flexibility, and feeling good, definitely keep foam rolling!

The peer-reviewed research on foam rolling and its underlying mechanisms is very new, but the results so far are promising. It appears foam rolling increases range of motion and muscle performance and diminishes perceived post-workout muscle soreness.

Here are 8 benefits of foam rolling, including the clinical research that's been conducted so far in support of each benefit.

MUSCLE AND TRIGGER POINT RELEASE

Adhesions and other damage- or overload-related stresses in fascia can lead to trigger points, which are very irritable points of taut muscle that are usually painful when compressed or stretched. They can cause restricted range of motion, localized muscular fatigue, and/or referred pain elsewhere. Some trigger points cause pain without being touched, like when you feel a muscle knot contributing to upper back pain even when you're not touching the area. Other trigger points are "latent," which means you don't notice them until they're touched directly (often during massage or foam rolling). Trigger points can refer pain to different areas. For example, a very tight point in the trapezius or levator scapulae muscles (both muscles of the upper back) can cause pain felt as a tension headache.

Localized compression of specific trigger points has long been considered useful in treating them. Recent research is supporting this idea. One study found that six repetitions of 30 seconds of compression on a trigger point with a "Backnobber" self-massage device, every other day for a week, decreased the research subjects' perceived sensitivity of the trigger points.[2]

IT BAND SYNDROME

The iliotibial (IT) band is a thick band of tissue that originates in the pelvis, runs along the outer length of the thigh, and crosses the knee to attach to the top part of the tibia (shin bone). IT band syndrome is one of the most common overuse injuries among runners, as well as other long-distance athletes such as cyclists.

IT band syndrome occurs when the IT band becomes inflamed or tight. This can cause pain anywhere along the IT band, but especially on the outer side of the knee. Often this pain is most pronounced when the heel strikes the ground while running.

Many people instinctively foam roll the IT band directly, because that's the area in which they feel pain. Registered massage therapist Karen Martens, however, is here to explain why this is not a good idea. Here is her advice:

I can't stress this enough: Stop rolling the IT band directly! The IT band becomes dysfunctional primarily for two reasons. First, it can become adhered to the structures underneath it, which are the vastus lateralis (one of the quadriceps muscles) and the biceps femoris (the main hamstring muscle). Second, the IT band can become dysfunctional when the gluteus medius—a muscle at the top and outer side of the hip—is no longer firing properly.

Rolling directly over the IT band only increases the adhesions between it and the muscles underneath it, making the situation

---

2   Gulick, D. T., Palombaro, K., & Lattanzi, J. B. (2011). Effect of ischemic pressure using a Backnobber II device on discomfort associated with myofascial trigger points. *Journal of Bodywork and Movement Therapies, 15*(3), p. 319-325.

worse. Instead, make sure to roll the most lateral (outside of the body) portion of the vastus lateralis and biceps femoris muscles, where they meet with the IT band. This will decrease the tension in the muscles themselves as well as any adhesions along the edge of the IT band, giving it a chance to start sliding and gliding as it's supposed to.

In addition to rolling these areas, I highly recommend rolling the glutes as well, most importantly the gluteus medius. When this muscle stops firing, the hip is no longer stable. This creates more work for the IT band, which then leads to adhesions as well as potential knee pain.

Anatomy Related to the IT Band

Iliotibial band (ITB): Runs down the outer thigh from the hip to just below the knee, and attaches to the tensor fasciae latae (TFL) at the hip.

Tensor fasciae latae (TFL): Small muscle on the outside of the hip that assists in hip stabilization and hip abduction (moving the femur, or thigh bone, outward to the side, as in taking the thighs apart).

Gluteus medius (also known as the glute med): Sits just behind the TFL on the hip. The glute med is a main hip abductor and hip stabilizer.

Vastus lateralis: The outermost quad muscle, runs underneath the ITB.

Biceps femoris: The outermost hamstring muscle, also runs underneath the ITB.

ITB problems include shortening, friction at the knee, and thickening (also called fasciitis), causing pain at the knee when it's really a problem in the hips. All these problems occur due to a weak or non-functioning glute med. The main reason the glute med is weak in many people is prolonged periods of sitting or inactivity.

When the glute med stops firing, the hip tends to "drop" on the weight bearing side, causing the knee to compensate medially or laterally in order to maintain alignment. This causes the ITB to "rub" or cause friction on the structures underneath it–the vastus lateralis and the biceps femoris.

In order to fix these problems, ensure you foam roll the glute med, TFL, vastus lateralis, and biceps femoris. [Karina's note: you'll find these muscles under the "Glutes," "Tensor Fasciae Latae," "Quads," and "Hamstrings" headings, respectively, in the self-myofascial release section of the foam rolling exercises in this book.]

In addition to foam rolling, strengthen the glute med and the TFL. While standing, feet hip width apart, bring one foot directly out to the side (abduction) without tilting your body or hips. Your hip bones should stay level at all times. A second way to perform this exercise is by lying on your side. The movement is the same: the leg is moving up and the outside of the foot moves toward the ceiling. Again, make sure you're not compensating by rolling the hips in any direction.

Step-downs are also helpful in re-training the glute med and the TFL. Standing on a low step with your hips aligned, slowly lower one foot off the step onto the ground, not allowing the hips to tilt throughout the entire movement. This works the side of your body that remains on the step.

Karen Martens, RMT

Physioworks, Vancouver, BC

MUSCLE RECOVERY AND DELAYED ONSET MUSCLE SORENESS (DOMS)

Among athletes and fitness professionals, foam rolling is a very common method of muscle recovery between workouts. Most people who exercise have at some point experienced muscle soreness from their workouts. This is especially common in people who strength train using weights, resistance bands, or bodyweight. When you exercise at a moderate to vigorous intensity, you're creating microscopic tears in your muscles. This is called exercise-induced muscle damage (EIMD). EIMD results in delayed onset muscle soreness (DOMS), the "good pain" you feel in your muscles in the day or two after a challenging workout. DOMS usually peaks between 24 and 48 hours after exercise. Muscle growth and strength increases happen while your muscles repair themselves in the days following your workout.

Massage is often used to treat DOMS. It's been shown to improve blood flow while decreasing perceived muscle soreness, inflammation, and cellular stress.[3] In one study, 20 male subjects with three or more years of strength training experience participated in testing sessions involving the weighted squat. Ten subjects performed foam rolling for 20 minutes after squatting heavy weights, and the other ten subjects didn't foam roll. Perceived muscle soreness at 24, 48, and 72 hours after testing was significantly lower among those who foam rolled, compared to those who didn't. Range of motion was also greatly increased in the foam rolling group.[4]

---

3   Button, D. C., & Behm, D. G. (April, 2014). Foam rolling: early study findings suggest benefits. Accessed May 27, 2014 at http://lermagazine.com/article/foam-rolling-early-study-findings-suggest-benefits.
4   Macdonald, G. Z., Button, D. C., Drinkwater, E. J., & Behm, D. G. (2014). Foam rolling as a recovery tool after an intense bout of physical activity. *Medicine & Science in Sports & Exercise, 46*(1), p. 131-142.

A yet-to-be-published study found that foam rolling, compared to the control condition, significantly decreased quadriceps muscle tenderness at 24 and 48 hours after the exercise intervention. It also substantially improved sprint time (at 24 and 72 hours), muscle power (at 24 and 72 hours), and dynamic strength-endurance (at 48 hours). The researchers concluded that foam rolling can be effective in reducing DOMS and its associated decreases in dynamic physical performance measures.[5]

Keep in mind that many of the studies described here have small sample sizes—sometimes 20 participants or less. This makes it difficult to extrapolate results to the rest of the population. There certainly is promising research that shows benefits to foam rolling, but what really matters is whether it works for you! The only way to know is to give it a try.

FLEXIBILITY AND MOBILITY

Flexibility and mobility are two separate, but related, concepts. Flexibility is part of mobility, but extreme flexibility is not needed for good mobility. Flexibility is defined as the range of motion in a joint or series of joints, or the ability of a muscle (or a group of muscles) to lengthen through a range of motion. Greater range of motion at a certain joint means having greater flexibility.

Mobility means being able to perform functional movement patterns without restrictions in the range of motion of those movements. Mobility takes into account more than flexibility, including joints, muscles crossing the joints, and motor control from the nervous system. Someone can be very flexible but can lack the coordination, strength, and/or balance required for great mobility.

---

5   Pearcey, G. E. P., et al. (2014). Effects of foam rolling on delayed onset muscle soreness and recovery of dynamic performance measures. *Journal of Athletic Training.* [In press.]

Both flexibility and mobility can be improved by using the foam roller. See the Flexibility and Mobility section of exercises of this book for detailed exercise instructions.

Fitness professionals usually differentiate between the benefits of stretching and the benefits of self-myofascial release by foam rolling, even though both methods can lead to an increase in range of motion. Stretching improves the *length* of your muscles, while foam rolling and other massage work adjusts the *tone* of your muscles. Ideally, in a well-rounded fitness program, you'd perform both stretching and soft tissue work such as foam rolling and/or massage.

Foam rolling seems to provide similar benefits in range of motion (a measure of flexibility) to static stretching[6, 7, 8] and massage.[9, 10] A clear advantage to using a foam roller compared to static stretching to increase range of motion is that stretching is often associated with decreases in athletic performance.[11, 12] No study has yet found a decrease in performance after foam rolling. In fact, there is some evidence that

6   Behm, D. G. & Kibele, A. (2007). Effects of differing intensities of static stretching on jump performance. *European Journal of Applied Physiology, 101*(5), p. 587-594.

7   Murphy, J. R., Di Santo, M. C., Alkanani, T., & Behm, D. G. (2010). Aerobic activity before and following short-duration static stretching improves range of motion and performance vs. a traditional warm-up. *Applied Physiology, Nutrition, and Metabolism, 35*(5), p. 679-690.

8   Power, K. et al. (2004). An acute bout of static stretching: effects on force and jumping performance. *Medicine & Science in Sports & Exercise, 36*(8), p. 1389-1396.

9   Huang, S. Y. et al. (2010). Short-duration massage at the hamstrings musculotendinous junction induces greater range of motion. *Journal of Strength and Conditioning Research, 24*(7), p. 1917-1924.

10   McKechnie, G. J. B., Young, W. B., & Behm, D. G. (2007). Acute effects of two massage techniques on ankle joint flexibility and power of the plantar flexors. *Journal of Sports Science and Medicine, 6*(4), p. 498-504.

11   Behm, D. G. & Chaouachi, A. (2011). A review of the acute effects of static and dynamic stretching on performance. *European Journal of Applied Physiology, 111*(11), p. 2633-2651.

12   Kay, A. D. & Blazevich, A. J. (2012). Effect of acute static stretch on maximal muscle performance: a systematic review. *Medicine & Science in Sports & Exercise, 44*(1), p. 154-164.

foam rolling can actually increase physical performance, while still increasing range of motion.[13]

One 2013 study investigated the effect of foam rolling on muscle activation and force, as well as range of motion.[14] Eleven physically active males were recruited for the study. Foam rolling the quadriceps muscle for two minutes significantly increased the knee joint range of motion, without decreasing muscle activation or force. The range of motion increased by 12.7% and 10.3% at two and ten minutes after foam rolling, respectively. The take-home message from this study is that foam rolling before a workout could be quite beneficial to your range of motion, and thus potentially your physical performance.

Another 2013 study found similar results. The study tested whether foam rolling the hamstring muscle group could increase flexibility among 15 amateur female soccer players.[15] The study authors note that hamstring injuries are among the most common injuries reported in professional football, so a protocol that could decrease this risk would be very valuable. The researchers used a common test to measure hamstring flexibility called the active lying knee extension test. If you were being tested, you'd lie supine (on your back) with your legs straight, resting on the floor. The test administrator would hold down your right leg to make sure it doesn't leave the floor, as you bend your left hip and knee at right angles. Now your thigh is vertical (perpendicular to the floor) and your lower leg is horizontal (parallel to the floor). Keeping your thigh vertical, you'd extend

---

13   Bradbury-Squires, D. J. et al. (2014). Roller massager application to the quadriceps increases knee joint ROM and neuromuscular efficiency during a lunge. *Journal of Athletic Training*. [In press.]

14   MacDonald, G. Z., et al. (2013). An acute bout of self-myofascial release increase range of motion without a subsequent decrease in muscle activation or force. *Journal of Strength and Conditioning Research, 27*(3), p. 812-821.

15   Sheffield, K. & Cooper, N. (2013). The immediate effects of self-myofascial release on female footballers. *SportEX Dynamics, 38*, p. 12-17.

your left knee as far as is comfortable, and the test administrator would measure the angle your knee creates. An angle of 5 to 15 degrees[16] is typically desirable. If your hamstrings are not very flexible, the angle would be greater. If you're really flexible, the angle would be smaller.

In the study with female soccer players, the researchers wanted to see whether the angle at the knee joint would decrease after foam rolling. The study found that, immediately after foam rolling the hamstring muscle, active knee extension test scores did indeed improve. This means hamstring flexibility significantly increased directly after foam rolling.

A new, yet-to-be-published study used a roller-massager stick (imagine a ridged rolling pin for your muscles) on the quadriceps muscle and found an increase in knee joint range of motion of 10% for the 20-second condition and 16% for the 60-second condition.[17]

Another study also using the roller-massager stick found a significantly greater range of motion at the ankle after rolling the back of the lower leg for three sets of 30 seconds.[18] Interestingly, muscle rolling improved muscular force, while static stretching decreased it. Both static stretching and muscle rolling increased ankle range of motion immediately and 10 minutes after the intervention.

The sit-and-reach test is a classic measure of hamstring flexibility. If you were doing the test, you'd sit on the floor with your legs straight out in front of you, feet together. Your feet would be flat against a surface such as a box. Then, with arms straight out in front of you, you'd reach toward your

---

16   www.exrx.net, accessed May 22, 2014. Active lying knee extension. http://www.exrx.net/Testing/FlexFunction/LyingKneeExtension.html
17   Bradbury-Squires, D. J. et al. (2014). Roller massager application to the quadriceps increases knee joint ROM and neuromuscular efficiency during a lunge. *Journal of Athletic Training.* [In press.]
18   Halperin, I., et al. (2014). Roller massager improves range of motion of plantar flexor muscles without subsequent decreases in force parameters. *International Journal of Sports Physical Therapy, 9*(1), p. 92-102.

toes as far as you can go, and the distance you reached would be measured. One study used this test before and after using a roller-massager on the hamstrings, and also included a control group that did not use the roller. Using the roller increased joint range of motion by 4.3% after rolling for only 5 or 10 seconds. There was a trend for the 10-second condition to provide an additional 2.3% range of motion increase, but this wasn't quite statistically significant. [19]

INCREASING PHYSICAL PERFORMANCE

Increasing flexibility and mobility, which appears to be a benefit of foam rolling seen in the research literature so far, could lead to increased physical performance over time. Studies that directly investigate the effect of foam rolling on physical performance, however, are few and far between. Most studies so far have been conducted in short-term settings, which means the potential long-term performance effects have not yet been studied. However, a few recent studies have supported the idea that foam rolling can enhance physical performance within a short-term context.

Previous studies have shown that static stretching before exercise can decrease performance, particularly for explosive movements such as sprints or vertical jumps.[20, 21] It appears that foam rolling has similar positive effects on joint range of motion compared to stretching, but has never been shown to decrease physical performance. In one study, in fact, foam

19   Sullivan, K. M., Silvey, D. B., Button, D. C., & Behm, D. G. (2013). Roller-massager application to the hamstrings increases sit-and-reach range of motion within five to ten seconds without performance impairments. *International Journal of Sports Physical Therapy, 8*(3), p. 228-236.

20   Fletcher, I. M. and Jones, B. (2004). The effect of different warm-up stretch protocols on 20 meter sprint performance in trained rugby union players. *Journal of Strength & Conditioning Research, 18*(4), p. 885-888.

21   Bradley, P. S., Olsen, P. D., & Portas, M. D. (2007). The effect of static, ballistic, and proprioceptive neuromuscular facilitation stretching on vertical jump performance. *Journal Strength & Conditioning Research, 21*(1), p. 223-226.

rolling lead to an 8.2% *increase* in maximal voluntary isometric contraction (a measure of muscle force) compared to static stretching, measured ten minutes after the intervention.[22] This increase in muscle force could be due to an increase in muscle temperature caused by friction, the release of myofascial restrictions, or the action of submaximal muscle contractions that may occur during foam rolling. This supports the idea that the mechanisms behind foam rolling may be more closely related to those of massage than to those of static stretching.[23]

A recent study published in the *Journal of Strength and Conditioning Research* set out to determine whether foam rolling increased athletic performance.[24] Thirteen men and 13 women of college age were tested on vertical jump height and power, isometric (also called static) muscle force, and agility after either foam rolling or performing a series of planking exercises. In addition to physical performance, fatigue, soreness, and exertion were also measured. Interestingly, there were no differences in physical performance between groups, which means foam rolling had no effect on performance. However, post-exercise fatigue was significantly lower for subjects who had performed foam rolling instead of planking. This could be due to the fact that planking may have been more physically rigorous than foam rolling. If this wasn't the case, reduced fatigue due to foam rolling after exercise may allow athletes to extend their training volume and training time, which would lead to increased performance over time. In an acute setting, where the study set-up was not longitudinal,

---

22   Halperin, I., et al. (2014). Roller massager improves range of motion of plantar flexor muscles without subsequent decreases in force parameters. *International Journal of Sports Physical Therapy, 9*(1), p. 92-102

23   Button, D. C., & Behm, D. G. (April, 2014). Foam rolling: early study findings suggest benefits. Accessed May 27, 2014 at http://lermagazine.com/article/foam-rolling-early-study-findings-suggest-benefits.

24   Healey, K. C. et al. (2014). The effects of myofascial release with foam rolling on performance. *Journal of Strength and Conditioning Research, 28*(1), p. 61-68.

foam rolling had no effect on performance. Since the sample size of this study was quite small, further research is required, using larger sample sizes and longer time frames.

CORE STRENGTH AND STABILITY

Your "core" isn't just your abs—it's also your lower back and pelvic region, including the hip abductors and adductors, hip flexors, lumbar spine, and pelvic floor. The diaphragm—the main muscle involved in breathing—is also considered part of the core.

Most people are more familiar with the term "strength" than the term "stability," even though we've probably all heard "stability" used in reference to core exercises by fitness class instructors, personal trainers, or other fitness professionals. Strength is our ability to exert force on physical objects by using our muscles. It's the state of being strong. Core strength, then, means having strong muscles in your abdominal and lower back region.

But what is core stability, exactly? In technical terms, core stability is "the ability to control the position and motion of the trunk over the pelvis to allow optimum production, transfer and control of force and motion to the terminal segment in integrated athletic activities."[25] Basically, it's the ability of the abdominal region, lower back, and pelvis to keep your body stable during movement. A stable core will allow you to maintain balance, prevent injury, and perform movements effectively.

Core strength and stability contribute to many aspects of a healthy, functioning body. Strong core muscles support proper posture and spinal alignment, which is important for everyday activity—from gardening to sitting at a desk, and from lifting weights to walking. A strong and stable core can prevent and decrease lower back pain, which is one of the most

---

25   Kibler, W. B., Press, J., & Sciascia, A. (2006). The role of core stability in athletic function. *Sports Medicine, 36*(3), p. 189-198.

common medical complaints among North Americans.[26] A strong and stable core also absorbs impact and transmits forces throughout the body in an efficient manner. For example, boxers need tremendous core strength and stability to efficiently transfer force from the legs to the arms while delivering a punch. Most sports (or any physical activity, for that matter) rely on strong and stable core muscles to carry out the required movements.

Many foam roller exercises are excellent for increasing core strength and stability. Due to the nature of the foam roller (it rolls!), your core muscles will be recruited to help you maintain your position and balance on the roller. Check out the Strength and Core Stability section in the exercise chapter of this book for a closer look at the movements you can perform on the foam roller to increase your core strength and stability.

DECREASING NEGATIVE IMPACTS OF PROLONGED SITTING

Many of us have mostly (or entirely) sedentary jobs, where we sit for 8 hours or more per day. Most of us also sit during our commutes to work. Even if we go for regular runs or work out at the gym consistently, most of our leisure hours are also spent sitting (e.g. eating meals, watching TV, browsing the Internet). We probably all know that this much sitting isn't good for us. Unfortunately, recent research is revealing that it's probably much worse for our bodies than we might think. While research into the benefits of physical activity is very robust and conclusive, examining the negative effects of sedentary lifestyles is a relatively new area of research.

Negative effects of prolonged sitting found so far in the research literature include increased risk for cardiovascular disease, cancer, and metabolic syndrome (a cluster of conditions that includes high blood sugar and

---

26   Hoy, D., et al. (2012). A systematic review of the global prevalence of low back pain. *Arthritis & Rheumatology, 64*(6), p. 2028-2037.

cholesterol levels, high blood pressure, and excess abdominal fat). Sitting for long periods of time seems to disrupt metabolic function, which can lead to decreased insulin sensitivity, decreased levels of high-density lipo-protein cholesterol (the "healthy" kind), and increased plasma triglyceride levels. One major reason why sitting can slow down metabolism is that the major muscle groups like the legs and back aren't contracting while we sit. Long-term sitting can also cause muscle imbalances and postural issues, which we'll address shortly. Some studies even find an association between prolonged sitting and death due to all causes!

Interestingly, research is showing that a few hours a week of moderate- to vigorous-intensity physical activity doesn't offset the nega-tive effects of prolonged sitting. Of course, regular physical activity is very important in its own right, as one of the most essential components of a healthy lifestyle. The point is that prolonged sitting is a risk factor on its own, regardless of how much or how often you exercise outside of sitting. Instead of increasing our physical activity levels outside of work (which is the most common arena for sedentary behavior), the solution seems to be minimizing sitting in the first place, while increasing overall movement throughout the day.[27]

One study fitted its participants with accelerometers (devices that measure movement, speed, and direction) that were worn during waking hours for 7 hours a day, 7 days in a row. The researchers measured interrup-tions in sedentary time for each participant. An interruption didn't have to be a long break like going for a walk. Even one step counted as a break in sedentary time. Increased breaks in sedentary time were associated with a lower waist circumference, lower body mass index, and more favourable triglyceride and plasma glucose levels. These beneficial effects were found

---

27   Levine, J. A. What are the risks of sitting too much? Accessed July 2, 2014. http://www.mayoclinic.org/healthy-living/adult-health/expert-answers/sitting/faq-20058005

independently of moderate- to vigorous-intensity physical activity and total sedentary time.[28] That means the number of breaks a participant took during sedentary time predicted waist circumference, BMI, triglyceride levels, and plasma glucose levels, regardless of their total physical activity levels and total sedentary time!

A 2012 study of more than 222,000 people aged 45 and older found that sitting for 11 or more hours per day increased the risk of death by 40%, regardless of overall physical activity levels. This association between prolonged sitting and all-cause mortality was consistent across the sexes, age groups, physical activity levels, and body mass index categories. The relationship also existed in both healthy participants and those with pre-existing cardiovascular disease or diabetes.[29]

Another study conducted two years earlier investigated adult men and their risk of dying from heart disease. Men who reported more than 23 hours per week of sedentary activity, including sitting at a work desk, watching TV, and riding in a car, had a 64% greater risk of dying from heart disease compared to those who reported less than 11 hours of sedentary activity for the week. This relationship remained even after controlling for variables such as total physical activity.[30]

As you can see from the research, the more breaks you can take during sedentary time and the more you can avoid sedentary time in the first place, the better off you'll be when it comes to your health. Keep in mind that each break doesn't have to take up much time. Even getting up from your chair briefly or standing to stretch is fine, as long as you do it

28   Healy, G. N. et al. (2008). Breaks in sedentary time: beneficial associations with metabolic risk. *Diabetes Care, 31*(4), p. 661-666.
29   Van der Ploeg, H. P., Chey, T., Banks, E., and Bauman, A. (2012). Sitting time and all-cause mortality risk in 222,497 Australian adults. *Archives of Internal Medicine, 172*(6), p. 494-500.
30   Warrens, T. Y. et al. (2010). Sedentary behaviours increase risk of cardiovascular disease mortality in men. *Medicine & Science in Sports & Exercise, 42*(5), p. 879-885.

regularly. Stand up, march in place, take a few steps back and forth, do a little dance. This isn't about working out more (which is positive in its own right but doesn't offset the effects of prolonged sitting). It's about creating pockets of physical activity throughout the day and giving your body a break from long-term sitting. Just as regular physical activity and a good diet are requirements for a long, disease-free life, so too is taking breaks from prolonged sitting. At the office, try to get up from your chair at least every hour (more often if you can). Take a brief walk during your lunch break, or at least eat your lunch and make your phone calls standing up.

If you want the most bang for your buck, why not foam roll a few times throughout the day? Not only will you be taking a break from being sedentary, but you'll also benefit your muscles, helping to reverse some of the negative effects of sitting for long periods of time.

Even though many negative effects of long-term sitting aren't mitigated by a few hours of physical activity per week, regular and consistent foam rolling may help you to treat and prevent spinal and postural problems associated with prolonged sitting. Sitting for long periods of time wreaks havoc on the spine. People who sit for long periods of time each day are more likely to suffer from herniated disks in the lumbar spine compared to people who don't sit as much.

Due to lots of sitting, we can lose the ability to properly rotate from the upper back—also called the thoracic spine area. When the muscles surrounding the thoracic spine lose their ability to rotate properly, other areas of the body have to compensate. Rotation then often happens in the cervical (neck) spine area, and/or the lumbar (lower back) spine area instead, which often leads to low back pain. These compensations don't just affect the back, however. Problems here can affect other joints, including the shoulders and knees.

Sitting for prolonged periods of time also decreases thoracic extension, which is the ability of the spine and muscles in the upper back area to extend in the direction of a person's back, or move to produce backward bending. In contrast, thoracic flexion is movement in the opposite direction, which is rounding the upper back or "slouching" forward. Poor thoracic extension can lead to a sub-par overhead position for the shoulders, a rounded upper back, and an increase in lumbar extension (lordosis, or an exaggerated curve in the lower back). The spine, seen from the side, naturally has curves in it to support the weight of the head and to absorb shock. Problems occur, however, when these natural curves are exaggerated and greater than normal. An excessive rounding of the upper back due to bad posture is called postural kyphosis. This leads to a "hunchback" appearance with the head jutting forward. Kyphosis is usually accompanied by muscle weakness, stiffness, and pain. If not corrected, these symptoms usually remain constant and often become progressively more severe over time.

Having impaired thoracic extension and rotation means having low thoracic mobility. Here's a simple test you can do yourself to assess your own thoracic mobility. Lie down on your back on the floor, with your knees bent and feet flat on the floor, about hip width apart. Make sure your entire back is touching the floor. This means you'll need to tighten your abdominal muscles to press your lower back into the floor. Maintaining this position with your back, lock your elbows and bring your arms straight toward the ceiling, shoulder width apart and palms facing each other. Now try to touch your wrists to the ground above your head, keeping your arms perfectly straight and your lower back completely pressed into the floor. If you need to arch your back in order to touch your wrists to the floor behind your head, if it's uncomfortable, or if you just can't do it, you likely have less than optimal mobility in your thoracic spine.

The foam roller is uniquely positioned to be very effective at minimizing negative effects of prolonged sitting. You can perform flexibility, mobility, strength, and stability exercises with a foam roller, which is a very well-rounded approach to fitness.

Many foam roller exercises focus on mobilizing the thoracic spine, which should be a priority if you discover you have low thoracic spine mobility, have a sedentary job, or otherwise spend a lot of time sitting. Working on mobilizing your thoracic spine will help to prevent associated problems if you don't currently have them, and it'll help to treat them if you do.

If you have a sedentary job, a brief foam rolling session after work can help to keep you feeling your best, "undo-ing" some of the damage your body experiences from sitting for long periods of time. Many people also like taking small foam rollers along when they travel, to treat travel induced muscle stiffness, and of course to help with muscle recovery from workouts. At home, try leaving your foam roller in a clearly visible spot in your living room. Instead of sitting on the couch while watching TV, foam roll your muscles! You'll feel much more refreshed than if you'd been sedentary on the couch.

DECREASING AND PREVENTING LOW BACK PAIN

Low back pain is one of the most common medical complaints across the globe. Estimates vary, but one meta-analysis of 165 studies from 54 countries found that about 23% of the population experiences lower back pain at some point within one month. Within a lifetime, up to 40% of the population experiences back pain.[31]

---

31   Hoy, D., et al. (2012). A systematic review of the global prevalence of low back pain. *Arthritis & Rheumatology, 64*(6), p. 2028-2037.

If you currently have low back pain, movements and exercises using a foam roller may be appropriate for you to decrease your pain. Certain movements using the foam roller are also effective at preventing lower back pain so you don't have to experience it in the first place. Make sure you check with a health and/or fitness professional to ensure you're doing what's right for you.

In many cases, low back pain can be caused by tightness in the upper back. It sounds counterintuitive, but if your upper back is tight, movements that are supposed to be executed by the upper back muscles are instead carried out by the lower back, causing pain and dysfunction over time. Movements such as the Thoracic Spine Extension or the Quadruped Thoracic Rotation (see the Flexibility and Mobility section of the exercise chapter of this book) may help to increase mobility in the upper back. For many people, increasing core strength and stability helps to alleviate and to prevent low back pain. Take a look at the Strength and Core Stability section of the exercise chapter for detailed exercise instructions.

NOTES ON FOAM ROLLING RESEARCH

Foam rollers have been used in physical therapy settings for many years. Clinical research in the area, however, is relatively new. Results so far are promising, but much more work is needed.

Most studies that have been conducted so far, like the ones described in this book, used small sample sizes. That means only about 20–and sometimes fewer–people participated in many of the studies. Often, the study participants were selected based on specific criteria, like being female soccer players, being aged 45 and older, or being male college students who have been training athletically for at least a year. This makes it difficult to generalize study results to the population as a whole. For example, foam rolling may increase muscle range of motion for young athletes who train regularly, but does it have the same effect for older, less active individuals? Preliminary results show that foam rolling likely benefits anyone, but we need more high quality research with much larger sample sizes to be sure.

Most foam rolling research conducted so far has studied foam rolling within a relatively short time frame, such as measuring athletic performance a few minutes after foam rolling, or measuring muscle range of motion before and after foam rolling for a few days or a week. Future research should include long-term studies of foam rolling, such as measuring the effect of 5 minutes of daily foam rolling over a number of months, or even years. At this point we can only assume that regular, consistent foam rolling over time will lead to greater results, but we need clinical research to be sure.

Numerous studies have found that foam rolling can improve range of motion, muscle performance, and post-workout recovery. It's still unclear which physiological mechanisms are at work, so further research should be conducted. Future research should also compare foam rolling to other modes of massage or bodywork, such as massage therapy or active release massage techniques.

CHAPTER 3:
HOW TO FOAM ROLL

BEFORE YOU START: SAFETY AND PREPARATION

Before you start using a foam roller regularly, make sure you get the go-ahead from a licensed fitness or health care professional, especially if you've recently experienced an injury. You need to ensure that foam rolling is safe for you. Most health professionals will discourage foam rolling for people who have chronic pain diseases, like fibromyalgia, and possibly also people who have intervertebral disc problems. If you're unable to support yourself on your arms and/or legs, foam rolling may not be for you. If you're injury free and just need a little more strength in order to assume the foam rolling positions, focus on regular resistance training for a few weeks in order to build up the strength necessary for foam rolling.

Once you get the OK from a qualified practitioner, I suggest you get personalized instruction on which foam roller exercises would benefit you, and which you may need to avoid. Why not bring this book with you to your appointment? It's best to know what you're trying to achieve with foam rolling, whether it's better movement quality, less day-to-day pain, improved physical performance, decreasing the negative effects of prolonged sitting, post-workout muscle soreness relief, or anything in between (or a combination of different goals). A fitness professional or physical therapist can help you to determine which specific foam roller exercises will be best suited to your goals.

Many foam roller moves involve lying on your back, so make sure you're comfortable in this position. The unstable nature of a foam roller may take a bit of getting used to if you've never used one before. To get acquainted with two of the basic body positions on the roller, first sit on the end of a roller, with the roller extending behind you. Then slowly roll your back down onto the roller, making sure your head is supported on the roller at the other end. The foam roller is now lengthwise along your spine, with your feet planted on the floor. This is the basic position for many core strengthening and stability moves. The other position is having the roller crosswise along your upper back, used for massaging certain muscle groups and for some flexibility and mobility work. Place the foam roller on the ground and sit about two feet in front of it. Lean back and place your upper back on the foam roller, so your torso is perpendicular to the roller. You can also get into this position by sitting on the foam roller, then carefully lowering your body toward the floor as you roll the roller toward your upper back. Just make sure you're not exerting very much pressure on the lower back as you roll upward from your glutes.

In certain foam rolling positions, especially those for your hamstrings and calves, you'll be supporting most of your bodyweight on your hands. Some people may experience shoulder and/or wrist discomfort. If you feel pain, first check to ensure your posture is correct. When supporting yourself on your hands, make sure your wrists are directly under your shoulders. You can also try gripping push-up bars of hexagonal dumbbells placed on the floor. This places your wrists into a more neutral position, without having your hand flat on the floor and wrists bent. You can also try removing one leg from the roller and placing it on the floor for some added support, so you're not supporting the majority of your bodyweight with your arms. If you're still experiencing shoulder or wrist discomfort in certain postures, try switching to a muscle roller stick instead of using the foam roller for those moves. See page 40 for an explanation of muscle roller sticks.

Remember, more pain isn't necessarily better, even if it's "good" pain like you'd feel during a deep tissue massage. Know that you can overdo it on a foam roller, so make sure you start slow, don't cause pain, and don't spend a prolonged period of time on a tender area. Spending excessive time on sore spots or trigger points can lead to bruising or tissue damage. Rather than spending 5 to 10 minutes at a time on a particularly sore spot, spend less time and perhaps roll more often throughout the day to prevent injuring your muscle tissue.

It's usually most comfortable and effective to wear workout clothing while foam rolling. You can foam roll any time throughout the day, but some positions on the roller require fabrics more flexible than jeans or office wear. You also don't want to wear something too heavy, like a thick sweater, which might minimize the effect of foam rolling. Foam rolling your upper back should be manageable in almost any clothing, while rolling the inner thigh muscles or completing strength or flexibility exercises on the foam roller almost certainly require workout attire.

Make sure you're always using your roller on a firm, non-slip surface that is free of obstacles. For any foam rolling exercise, including flexibility, strength, or massage, try to focus on proper breathing. Especially for movements that require heightened effort, you may find yourself holding your breath. Try to avoid this! Holding your breath while working out can rapidly spike your blood pressure, decrease available oxygen in your body, and make you feel dizzy or faint. Concentrate on taking regular, deep breaths instead.

When your muscles are sore a day or two after a workout, should you foam roll? The simple answer is yes, assuming the soreness doesn't impact your ability to maintain good form while foam rolling. If you're so sore you can't hold yourself up, it's probably best to take another rest day before foam rolling. Many people find that foam rolling when their muscles are sore actually helps those muscles to feel less pain (perhaps due to increased blood flow to the area). So, as long as you can maintain proper posture and form while rolling, go for it even when you're sore from a challenging workout.

Once you've completed your foam rolling session, there's really no elegant way to come off of a foam roller! Just carefully roll to the side and slide off.

HOW AND WHEN TO FOAM ROLL

If you've never foam rolled before, here's how it works. The basic idea is that you use your own bodyweight on a foam roller to exert pressure on your soft tissue. You'll likely need to use considerable core strength in order to hold certain positions, so foam rolling often doubles as core-strengthening work (and you can perform dedicated core strength exercises as well, such as the ones in this book). In order to roll areas such as the hamstrings or calves, you'll need to support much of your bodyweight on your arms, which means you'll require a certain level of upper body strength. The more you foam roll, the more intuitive and less physically demanding it becomes (and the less pain you'll feel in the muscles you're rolling).

Roll a muscle group on the roller, slowly, until you feel a "trigger point." You may have heard the term "muscle knot" used to describe these as well. You'll know you've hit one when you feel it! When you hit one of these trigger points, stop rolling and rest on the foam roller for about 20 seconds, in an effort to release the muscle knot. Make sure to breathe smoothly and try to relax the muscle in question. Foam rolling is typically a combination of slowly rolling along a muscle, and holding a static position to apply pressure to a particular spot without moving. When foam rolling, make sure you apply pressure to just your muscles, rather than your joints or bones.

The more of your body that is in contact with the ground, the less intense pressure you'll feel on a particular muscle group. Let's say you're rolling your left hamstring muscle (see page 77 for a photo and description). If you're making contact with the ground with both feet and both hands, there will be minimal pressure on your hamstring. If you lift your right leg off the roller, more weight will be placed upon your left leg on the roller, making the massage more intense.

Since you're essentially massaging yourself, likely without the direction of a physical therapist or other health professional, you'll need to ensure you're using the appropriate amount of pressure. People with lower muscle density may be more likely to injure themselves.

Most health and fitness professionals caution that rolling your lower back—also called the lumbar spine region—is not a good idea. Placing your lower back along the foam roller exaggerates its curvature (also called lordosis), which can put excess pressure on the lower discs of the spine. Also, there would be few thick muscles between the foam roller and your spine, which needs support and protection.

As with many things in health and fitness, there's no universal agreement from professionals about when you should roll (e.g. before a workout, after a workout, the day after lifting weights), how often to roll, or how long your foam rolling session should last. Many fitness professionals, including myself, use foam rolling with their clients as part of regular workouts. Some use rolling prior to a workout as part of a dynamic warm-up, and others roll after workouts to potentially decrease Delayed Onset Muscle Soreness (DOMS). In a typical one-hour personal training session, most fitness coaches typically allow 5 to 10 minutes for foam rolling.

You can foam roll any time you like! I have one in my living room to use a few times a day as I pass by it. Based on my own athletic training and goals, I most often use the foam roller directly after a back or leg workout, and to increase the mobility in my thoracic spine area. Make sure you work with a professional (e.g. physiotherapist) to determine the most effective use of a foam roller for you, what you should focus on, and how often to roll.

CREATING A FOAM ROLLING PROGRAM

Designing a foam roller program or routine for yourself is a bit different from designing standard gym workouts. Unless you're doing strength-based moves, set and repetition numbers are generally not used in foam rolling, because so many of the movements involve static stretches or a few slow, controlled movements. Perfect posture is much more important than the number of reps you complete. Think quality over quantity!

It's best to work with a professional fitness coach or physiotherapist (depending upon your particular goals) to create a comprehensive foam rolling program that will most benefit you. After working with a professional to set up your program and coach you through the movements using correct form, it'll be up to you to listen to your body. It will tell you which particular muscles are tight, how much pressure to use on the roller, and whether you're using the correct form for each movement.

Your foam rolling program may differ from day to day depending upon your physical activity type and intensity level. If you focus on squats or deadlifts at the gym one day, for example, your lower body will likely need the most attention (rolling the glutes, quads, hamstrings, and calves). If you swim the next day, you might benefit most from rolling the lats and upper back, as well as stretching the shoulder and chest muscles.

It's important to know your goals before creating a foam rolling program. Are you looking to improve your athletic performance? Decrease day-to-day muscle pain? Rehabilitate an injury? Reduce exercise-related muscle soreness? Each goal will involve different foam roller exercises. The exercises in this book are divided into three sections: self-myofascial release (massage), flexibility and mobility, and strength and core stability. You could combine several of the strength exercises to create a standalone workout, or you could use a few foam roller movements to supplement your existing workouts (which is what I recommend). For example, add a few foam roller core exercises to your existing core routine to challenge your muscles in a new way.

The most common approach for post-workout foam rolling is to target the muscle groups you focused on during your workout, starting with the largest muscle groups and then moving to smaller muscle groups. At any time (post-workout or not), you can perform a "full body scan" by rolling all the major muscle groups, such as your upper back, glutes, hamstrings, and quads. Then go back and work on the smaller muscle groups, especially those that feel like they need extra attention, such as the triceps, pectorals, calves, piriformis, etc. You may find a tennis or lacrosse ball effective for working some of the smaller muscle groups, such as the pecs and piriformis.

OTHER TECHNIQUES FOR SELF-MYOFASCIAL RELEASE

Other implements are often used for self-myofascial release, including muscle rollers like "The Stick" (like a rolling pin for your muscles), or dense balls like tennis balls, lacrosse balls, or balls made specifically for trigger point massage. Sometimes, depending upon the muscle group in question, using a smaller implement is more comfortable. For example, foam rolling the chest muscles is an awkward position for some people, so using a tennis or lacrosse ball can be a better alternative. The idea is the same as foam rolling: roll slowly over muscles, pausing on trigger points.

Muscle stick

Using a muscle roller stick may be more comfortable for you if you find certain muscle groups difficult to foam roll, like the outside of your lower legs, or your calves. Muscle sticks are also much more portable than foam rollers, which makes them perfect for travel. Check out www.thestick.net for an example. You generally don't get as much pressure on your muscles from using a stick compared to a foam roller, but it's easier to adjust the level of pressure when you're using a muscle stick compared to a foam roller.

Imagine rolling back and forth over your muscles with a rolling pin. That's essentially what you do with a muscle stick. (By all means, use the rolling pin from your kitchen!) Muscle roller sticks come in a variety of lengths and shapes. They're typically smaller in diameter compared to a rolling pin, and many have separate rolling spindles to better contour to your muscles.

Just like foam rolling, you use the stick to roll back and forth across your muscles in an effort to decrease soreness and tension. I find the muscle stick to be useful during desk work, because I don't even have to get up from my chair to use it! The downside is you have to get someone else to roll your upper back for you, which is something you can easily do yourself on a foam roller.

Tennis ball

Using a tennis ball can be very effective at releasing muscle tension. I find tennis balls are great for getting at very specific areas, like a particular muscle knot. Often we don't know about muscle knots until we find them while foam rolling! I suggest foam rolling all major muscle groups, and if you find small areas of tension or concentrated muscle knots, try using a tennis ball on those areas.

For tension in your back, stand against a wall with the tennis ball wedged between your back and the wall. Find the muscle knot you want to work on, and press your back into the ball. You can move around in little circles, or side to side—whatever you find feels good and releases tension.

For tension in your lower body, like glutes, hamstrings, or hips, sit or lie with the tennis ball under the muscle group in question, using your hands on the floor to take some of the weight off if necessary. Use your bodyweight to press into the ball. You can hold it stationary if you like, or move around from side to side. If your muscles are really tight, this can be quite painful! (But of course, it feels great once you're done.)

One area that is very tight in many people but isn't conducive to foam rolling is the bottoms of the feet. People who spend a lot of time standing or athletes who do a lot of jumping often experience tight plantar muscles on the bottoms of the feet. This area is easy to release using a tennis ball: just place the ball under one foot and roll in circles, side-to-side, or hold a stationary position on a particularly tight spot. If the muscles on the bottoms of your feet are very tight, you may want to start by rolling them on a tennis ball while seated. If you want more pressure, try it while standing upright, holding on to a stable object (such as a wall) for balance.

CHAPTER 4:
COMPLEMENTARY PRACTICES
FOR MUSCLE RECOVERY

As beneficial as foam rolling can be, keep in mind that it's not the whole story when it comes to recovering, training, and restoring your muscles and tissues. If you're not supporting your foam rolling routine with other basic elements of muscle recovery, you may hinder your results. Make sure you're eating a nutrient-dense diet, getting adequate sleep each night, and staying hydrated to ensure you're fully recovering your muscles from an active lifestyle.

Muscle recovery is just as important as physical activity; they go hand-in-hand when it comes to taking care of your body and achieving your fitness goals. By focusing on both exercise and recovery, you'll be getting the most out of your healthy lifestyle.

When you work out at a challenging intensity, you're creating microscopic tears in your muscle fibers. Don't worry, that's a good thing! (Unless you overdo it, of course.) This means your muscles need time between workouts to repair themselves. It's this between-workout time during which your muscles rebuild and gain density and strength. Your workout may last only 45 minutes, but it's what you do in the next 48 hours that can help or hinder getting the results you want. The general rule for weight training is to leave 48 hours between training the same muscle group. You could, for example, complete a full body circuit on Mondays and Fridays, or even on Mondays, Wednesdays, and Fridays. Or you could train upper body on Mondays, lower body on Tuesdays, upper body on Thursdays, and lower body on Fridays. There are countless "training splits" as the fitness nuts all call them—just find something that works both for your schedule and lifestyle, and lets each muscle group rest for at least 48 hours.

With cardio activities such as running or swimming, there's less of a consensus among fitness professionals as to how long muscles take to recover. If you're training regularly, keep tabs on how your body feels and whether it's telling you it needs rest. Take at least one day off from intense exercise each week, and try to mix up your activities so you're not always doing the same thing.

TAKE A REST DAY

A rest day means a day without intense exercise in order to give your body enough time to recover from regular training. Rest days are appropriate for you if you work out at a moderate-to-high intensity 4 to 6 times per week. Someone who works out once a week for 10 minutes does not need designated rest days. But someone training on most days of the week at a high intensity most certainly needs at least one rest day per week.

ACTIVE RECOVERY

If you regularly work out at a high intensity, active recovery days are often helpful. They're especially useful for those crazy fitness nuts who just can't deal with a day that involves no workout. In contrast to a rest day–where you're not doing any physical activity–active recovery means engaging in a low-intensity activity that differs from your regular workout activities.

For example, if you're a serious swimmer, your active recovery day might be going for an easy 20-minute bike ride. If you lift weights at the gym regularly, your active recovery might be going for a walk. The idea is to do a very light, low-impact activity for a short period of time. Active recovery is a good way to relax and to increase blood circulation. Increased circulation is thought to improve muscle recovery.[32]

---

32   Micklewright, D. P., R. Beneke, V. Gladwell, & M. H. Sellens. (2003). Blood lactate removal using combined massage and active recovery. *Medicine & Science in Sports & Exercise, 35*(5), p. S317

MASSAGE

Massage (via massage therapy or sports massage) is an excellent way to recover your muscles and leave them feeling much less sore and stiff. You'll also increase immune function,[33] circulation, and joint mobility while you're at it. Massage is a great method of preventing problems in the first place, including muscle knots, tension headaches, and various forms of injury. Most serious athletes have regular massages as part of their muscle recovery plans. A qualified massage therapist will be better able to focus on precisely the muscles in your body that require work, compared to foam rolling on your own. Foam rolling is still very important, of course—in part because it's so accessible—but ideally you'd use foam rolling to "fill in the gaps" between seeing a massage practitioner on a regular basis.

Regular massages can be quite a financial investment that some are unable or unwilling to make. For the low cost of a foam roller and its potential benefits, it's certainly a good option and is better than doing no soft tissue work at all! More research is needed to compare foam rolling with other techniques and to better understand its benefits. Do keep in mind that foam rolling likely does not replace the bodywork you'd get with a qualified massage therapist or physiotherapist. Even though foam rolling is often seen as a substitute for massage, foam rolling offers only compression of the body's tissues. Massage has the added benefit of also being able to separate layers of tissue from each other. For example, it's generally not recommended to foam roll the IT band (running along the outer thigh from the hip to the knee) or the lower back. However, these areas can be safely manipulated through massage, using different techniques.

33   Rapaport, M. H., Schettler, P., & Bresee, C. (2010). A preliminary study of the effects of a single session of Swedish massage on hypothalamic-pituitary-adrenal and immune function in normal individuals. *Journal of Alternative and Complementary Medicine, 16*(1), p. 1079-1088.

STRETCHING

Stretching directly after a workout can help your muscles to relax and to release tension. The clinical research jury is still out as to whether stretching can help to prevent muscle soreness in the days following a workout, but many people who work out regularly claim that it does. Make sure that you stretch when your muscles are warm, such as right after completing your workout, or after taking a hot shower. Stretching cold muscles–like at the beginning of a workout–can increase your risk of tears, strains, and pulls. It's also been shown to decrease physical performance.

Make sure that your stretching sessions are pain free. Stretch slowly, relax your muscles, and only go so far as to feel a pulling, and perhaps a very slight burning sensation, in the muscle(s) you're stretching. If you stretch too far and cause pain, your muscles' defense mechanisms will kick in, in an effort to prevent injury. Muscles try to protect themselves by contracting, which is the opposite effect of the one you want from stretching.

Static stretching involves holding a stretch in the same position for a period of time, like sitting on the floor with your legs straight in front of you, reaching toward your toes with your hands to stretch the hamstrings. Dynamic stretching moves a particular muscle group through its entire range of motion in a fluid manner, which means you're moving during the stretch. Examples of dynamic stretches are making circles with your arms (mobilizing the shoulder joint), or swinging one leg back and forth from the front of your body to the back while standing on the opposite foot (affecting the hip joint). Both static and dynamic stretches have benefits; work with a qualified fitness professional to ensure you're getting the most benefits from each.

Stretching has many of the same benefits of yoga (not surprisingly, since they're both based on increasing flexibility), including increasing range of motion, preventing injury, and decreasing pain from muscle tightness.

YOGA

Research is beginning to support the effectiveness of yoga in decreasing delayed onset muscle soreness (DOMS).[34] DOMS is the soreness you feel in the day or two after a particularly challenging or new-to-you workout. Many of my personal training clients swear by yoga as an effective tool in decreasing their muscle soreness between workouts with me at the studio.

Yoga is also great for increasing flexibility and preventing injury. Many of us don't stretch for long enough (or at all!) after a workout to see any flexibility improvements over time. Yoga is a great way to get a healthy dose of flexibility and range of motion training. Also, many people find yoga more interesting than holding static stretches at the gym after a workout.

If you don't yet do yoga regularly, give it a try as a cross-training tool for your preferred physical activities. My two main activities are weight lifting and swimming, but I use yoga once a week to stretch and recover my muscles.

SLEEP

Getting enough sleep is one of the most important things you can do to ensure your muscles recover and get stronger after a workout. During deep sleep stages, your pituitary gland releases growth hormone that facilitates muscle repair and tissue growth. Growth hormone deficiency often leads to an increased risk for obesity, decreased muscle mass, and a lowered capacity for exercise.[35]

The exact relationship between exercise and sleep is still unclear, but a host of research studies have found a connection between sleep deprivation and decreased performance and recovery. Inadequate sleep is linked

34   Boyle, C. A., et al. (2004). The effects of yoga training and a single bout of yoga on delayed onset muscle soreness in the lower extremity. *Journal of Strength and Conditioning Research, 18*(4), p. 723-729.
35   Miller, B. (2010). *Sleep and muscle recovery.* http://www.livestrong.com/article/155363-sleep-muscle-recovery

to having low energy levels and increased levels of the hormones that break down muscle,[36] which is not something you want if you're looking to get–and keep–a lean body and a healthy metabolism!

Sleep is a prime time for the cells in our bodies to build new proteins (also known as protein synthesis).[37] Because protein is the building block of muscle, make sure you get your beauty sleep to keep your muscles healthy and functioning well.

Every person has his or her own sleep needs. There's no "gold standard" ideal amount of sleep to get each night, although most health authorities recommend between 7 and 9 hours per night. You may need to do some experimentation to find your optimal sleep length. If you're waking up well rested each morning, it's a sign that you're getting enough sleep.

Not sure how much sleep you need? You can find out, but you need about 2 weeks of a very flexible schedule. Perhaps you can take a sleep vacation! Go to bed at the same time every night, and don't set an alarm. Just wake up naturally. You might sleep for longer than normal the first few nights if you're chronically sleep deprived and need to catch up on sleep, but take note of what time you wake up during the second week. You'll likely wake up at a similar time each morning, at which point you've discovered the amount of sleep your body needs.

For an easy 5-minute test of reaction time, which can be an indicator of whether or not you're getting enough sleep, search for Harvard's "How Awake Are You?" online test.

Many of us are chronically sleep deprived. Here are 9 tips to help you get the sleep your body needs:

36   Datillo, M., et al. (2011). Sleep and muscle recovery: Endocrinological and molecular basis for a new and promising hypothesis. *Medical Hypotheses*, 77 (2), 220-222.
37   National Institutes of Health; National Institute of Neurological Disorders and Stroke (2007). Brain basics: understanding sleep. http://www.ninds.nih.gov/disorders/brain_basics/understanding_sleep.htm#for_us

How to Get Enough Sleep

- Keep a consistent sleep schedule. This means going to bed and waking up at the same time every day, including weekends and holidays. If you're getting enough sleep each night, this is easier than it might sound. I go to bed between 9:30 and 10:00 p.m. each night, and get up between 5:30 and 6:00 a.m. every morning. Not only has this schedule helped me to get enough sleep each night (my sleep cycle isn't disrupted by sleeping in), but I also happen to really enjoy mornings, so I feel I get the most out of each day. Nothing like coming home on a Sunday morning having already eaten two breakfasts, worked out, and gone grocery shopping, to find my husband still sleeping!

- Try to minimize sleep-disrupting activities a few hours before bed. These include high-concentration activities, high intensity exercise, and watching TV.

- Limit light exposure at night, including sunlight, indoor lighting, and screens. Try the "f.lux" app that changes the color of your screen display (for Windows, Macs, iPhone, and iPad) based on the time of day. When the sun sets in your corner of the world, the f.lux app makes your computer or phone screen look like your indoor lighting. When the sun comes up in the morning, it changes your screen back to its normal colors. Various research studies have found that "blue light" from screens may disrupt our sleep. By using an app like f.lux, you're minimizing your screen's blue light.

- Have a bedtime routine so that you can get into "sleep mode" before hitting the sack. This tells your body to start winding down.

- Avoid caffeine, alcohol, nicotine, and other substances that interfere with sleep.

- Don't have a clock visible while you're trying to fall asleep. Watching the clock while you're trying to fall asleep will probably make you feel stressed that you're not falling asleep, which won't help your efforts!
- Keep tabs on your food intake. Going to bed either really hungry or really full can make it difficult to fall–and stay–asleep.
- Invest in a good quality mattress and pillow set. Spending some decent money on a great mattress was one of the best investments my husband and I have made so far! We noticed an immediate improvement in sleep quality, which affected how alert we feel during the day.
- Make sure your room is comfortable for sleep: cool, dark, quiet, and devoid of clutter. Make use of blackout curtains and/or earplugs if you need them.

CHAPTER 5:
FOAM ROLLER EXERCISES

The exercises in this book are grouped into three sections: Self-Myofascial Release, Flexibility and Mobility, and Strength and Core Stability. Based on your health and fitness goals, you may draw upon exercises from all three categories, or you may need to focus on one category in particular.

Self-myofascial release is the most common use for foam rolling, whereby you slowly roll along various muscle groups to release tension and muscle "knots." The Flexibility and Mobility section is comprised of exercises that will increase the range of motion of your muscles (flexibility), and improve the ability of your muscles and joints to move through a range of motion with no restrictions (mobility). Exercises in the Strength and Core Stability section work to improve the strength of muscles throughout the body, with a special focus on core strength. Because the foam roller provides an unstable surface, your core muscles will need to work to keep your body stable during movement (the definition of core stability). A stable core is important for everything from preventing injury and low back pain, to performing your best during athletic activity, to having correct posture and spinal alignment.

FLEXIBILITY & MOBILITY

Increasing your flexibility and mobility is one of the cornerstones of any fitness program. You'll be able to perform physical movements with a lower risk of injury and a greater range of motion. Some exercises in this section are static, or non-movement based, while others are dynamic and include movement. Make sure you ease slowly into each stretch, avoiding any "bouncing" movements, which can lead to injury.

Chest

Tight pectoral (chest) muscles are common in people with sedentary jobs. When this muscle group becomes too tight, it can pull the shoulders forward, leading to potential shoulder injuries and a forward slumped appearance. This position on the foam roller stretches the pectoral muscles to help return them to normal function.

Lie lengthwise on the foam roller with your tailbone at one end and your head at the other. Bend your knees and place your feet flat on the floor. Straighten your arms and bring them to 90 degrees from your body, palms facing the ceiling. Rest your arms on the floor and relax your chest and shoulder muscles.

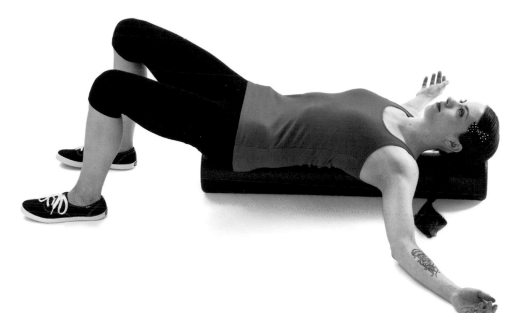

Shoulder drops

Release tension from your shoulders and upper back with this dynamic move.

Lie lengthwise on the foam roller with your tailbone at one end and your head at the other. Bend your knees and place your feet flat on the floor. Reach toward the ceiling with both arms straight (perpendicular to the floor), with palms facing each other. Now reach your right hand toward the ceiling, lifting your right shoulder blade off the roller. Then drop the right shoulder blade back onto the roller as low as you can. Imagine that you're hugging the roller with your shoulder blade. Then return to the starting position and repeat on the left side. You can also perform this exercise lifting and dropping both shoulder blades at the same time.

As you reach toward the ceiling, make sure your neck muscles aren't tightening and make sure you keep your head in contact with the foam roller.

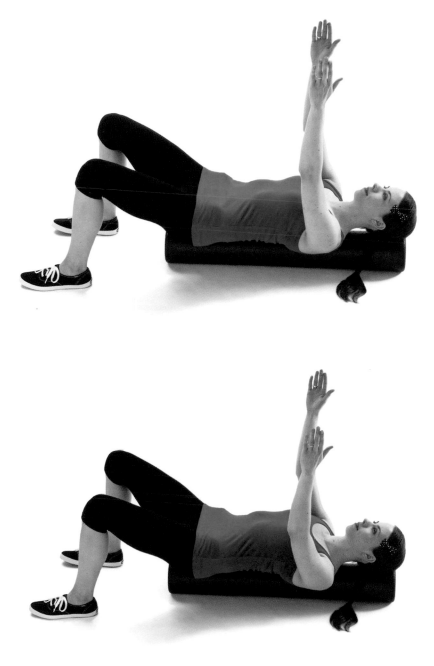

Thoracic spine extension

Improve your posture by increasing the mobility in your thoracic spine (the upper back area). Doing this can prevent rounding your shoulders from poor posture, especially if you have a sedentary job.

Place the foam roller crosswise under your upper back. Bend your knees and place your feet flat on the ground. Place your hands behind your head and move your elbows toward each other as far as you can. Slowly lean backward, dropping your head toward the floor. Slowly roll back up to the starting position, and repeat the move.

Make sure you keep your abdominals tightened and your pelvis in a neutral position so you don't excessively arch your lower back.

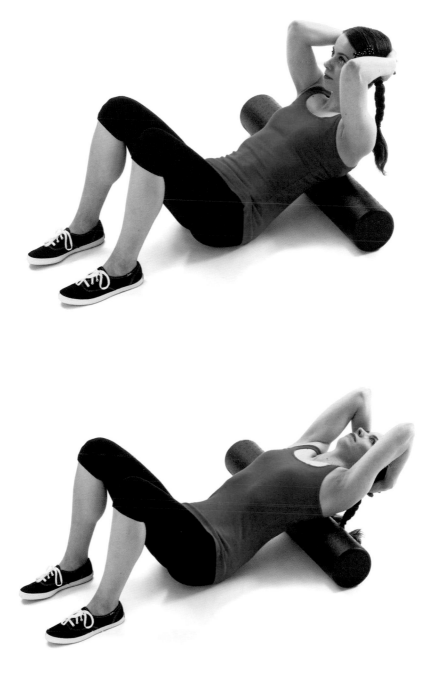

Quadruped thoracic rotation

This move increases mobility in the thoracic spine region (the upper back).

Kneel with your knees directly below your hips, and wrists directly below your shoulders. Place the foam roller lengthwise along the right side of your body. Keep your back as flat as possible, and ensure your weight is evenly distributed between both legs and arms. Place the back of your left hand on the roller, behind your right arm. Engage your abdominals. Reach your left hand away from your body, rolling the roller along the floor.

Make sure your hips don't rotate and that you keep a flat back throughout.

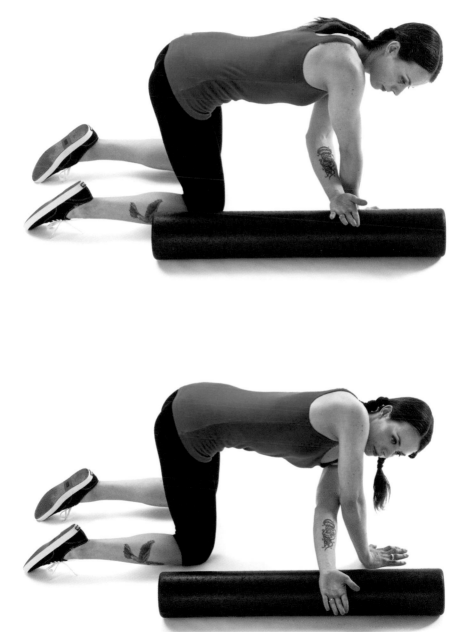

T-spine rotations

This is another exercise to mobilize your thoracic spine (also called the "T-spine").

Lying on your back, place one foam roller under your neck to support your head. Roll slightly to your left to place your right knee and lower leg on another foam roller placed by your left side. Straighten your left arm, resting it on the floor at a 90-degree angle to your body. Reach your right arm toward the ceiling, keeping it straight. Exhale and slowly reach your right arm to the right side, rotating the back of your right shoulder toward the floor. Make sure your right knee and lower leg maintain contact with the foam roller throughout this movement. Slowly return to the start position and repeat the move.

If you feel this exercise more in your lower back than your upper back, move your knee closer to your chest.

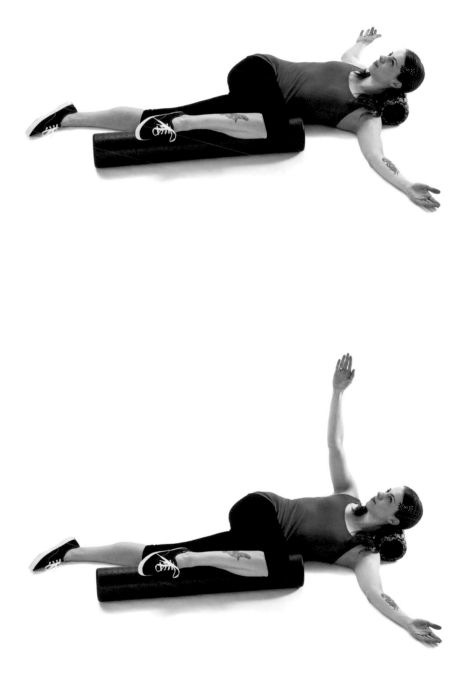

Cat stretch

This is a deep stretch for the latissimus dorsi (the "lats," the largest and widest muscle in the back), which in this stretch you'll most likely feel just under the armpits. This move also stretches the shoulders. Depending upon your level of mobility, it can be quite intense. Roll slowly and take your time!

Start by kneeling on the floor (using a mat if you like) with the foam roller in front of you. Rest your wrists or fingertips on the foam roller, with most of your weight supported by your knees and lower legs. Slowly roll the roller forward and away from your body, keeping your arms straight throughout the movement. Some of your weight will transfer from your knees to your upper body as you roll. Extend as far as is comfortable, hold, then return to the start position.

Make sure you ease slowly into this posture, especially if you're trying it for the first time, and avoid this move if you feel pins and needles in your hands or arms.

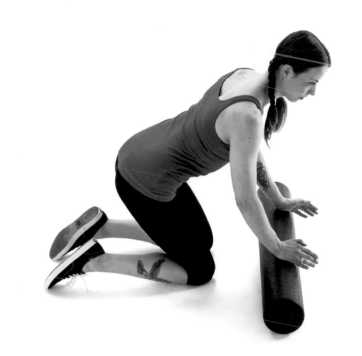

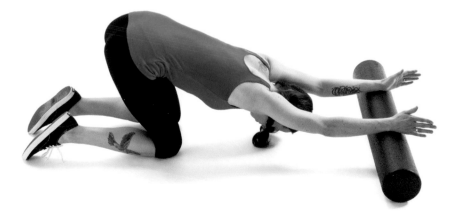

Single arm raises

This move stretches the pectoral muscles and increases range of motion at the shoulder joint.

Lie supine on the foam roller, with your tailbone at one end and your head at the other. Place your feet on the floor, hip width apart, and rest your arms by your sides. Raise your left arm toward the ceiling, making sure your left shoulder blade and your lower back are in contact with the roller at all times. Bring your arm above and behind your head to feel the stretch, hold for a few counts, and then slowly return your arm to the start position. Repeat on the right side.

Keep your abdominal muscles engaged throughout the exercise, keep the roller as stable as possible, and try to relax your pectoral muscles as you bring your arm overhead.

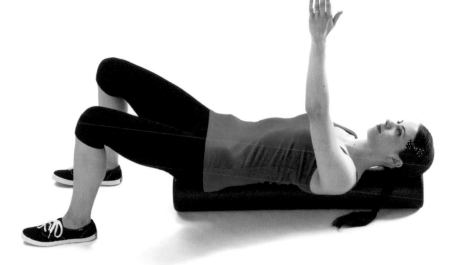

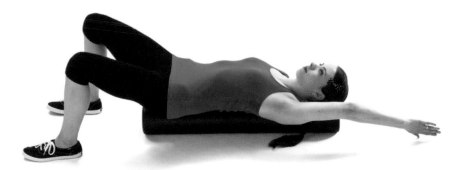

Hip flexor and psoas stretch

Tight hip flexor muscles are common in people who have postural problems. They can contribute to a forward tilting pelvis, which leads to a host of other problems like lower back pain. This foam roller exercise that stretches your anterior hip muscles (the hip flexors and the iliopsoas) is great to do after a long day of sitting, or after a lower body workout.

Start with the foam roller sideways, under your pelvis, so your body is perpendicular to the roller. Bend your knees and place your feet on the floor, hip width apart. You'll be resting on your upper back and head. Engage your abdominals, and raise your right knee to hug it into your chest. Then slide your left foot along the floor until your leg is straight, heel still on the floor. Keep your abdominals engaged throughout in order to prevent your back from arching. In other words, try to maintain a slight posterior tilt of the pelvis as you extend your left leg along the floor. Hold this position, then slide your left foot back to the start position and repeat on the other side.

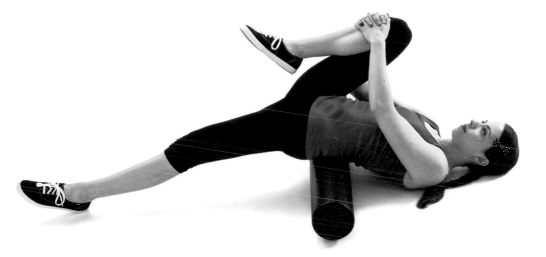

Camel pose

Camel pose in yoga stretches the front of the body, from the quads into the torso, including the chest and shoulders. Many people find the camel pose to be challenging, if not impossible, if done with the lower legs resting on the floor. This variation elevates the heels, which makes the move easier to perform.

Begin in a kneeling position, with your ankles resting on the foam roller behind you. Lean back slightly and place your hands on your heels or ankles. Keep your chest out and squeeze your shoulder blades together. Hold the pose for a few breaths, then release.

If you have lower back problems, make sure you get the go-ahead from a qualified health professional before you attempt this stretch.

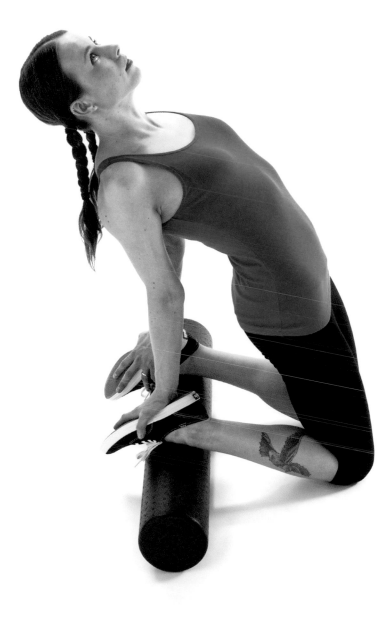

SELF-MYOFASCIAL RELEASE

You're likely most familiar with this collection of foam roller moves. It's the "classic" use of the foam roller: to massage muscle groups in an effort to decrease muscle tightness and ease muscle "knots." Typically, foam rolling is a combination of slowly rolling along a muscle, and holding a position to apply pressure to a particular knot or trigger point without moving. When foam rolling, make sure you apply pressure to only your muscles, rather than your joints or bones.

Hamstrings

Foam rolling your hamstrings may be especially beneficial after engaging in lower body-intensive sports like soccer or football. It may also prevent delayed onset muscle soreness (DOMS) in this muscle group after performing deadlifts or other hamstring-dominant weight lifting exercises.

Sit on the foam roller, with the roller placed sideways under your glutes. Place your hands on the floor behind you, hands facing forwards or to the side. With straight legs, lean onto your hands and roll the foam roller under your hamstrings, feet leaving the ground. Slowly roll the roller backwards and forwards along the hamstrings muscle. If you'd like more pressure, raise one leg so more weight is on the leg left on the roller.

Try to keep good posture throughout, with your head in alignment with your spine.

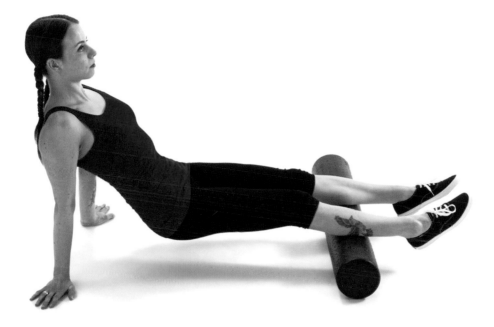

Quadriceps

Many runners have tight quadriceps (a.k.a. quad) muscles, which can set them up for injuries and sub-par performance. Rolling your quads could also be useful after engaging in activities such as cycling, hiking, or training your lower body by lifting weights (e.g. squats).

From a kneeling position, place the foam roller under your legs, with most of your bodyweight supported by your forearms on the floor. Roll slowly along the quadriceps muscles to release tension. You can lean from side to side to target the inner and outer portions of the quadriceps muscles.

Try to prevent your back from arching (anterior pelvic tilt) through-out the movement, and keep your head in line with your spine. Make sure to roll just the quadriceps muscles, and not the knees.

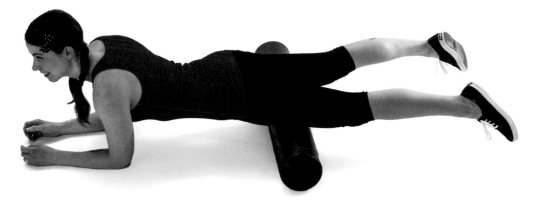

Calves

The calves may not be a muscle group we immediately think of when we think about foam rolling, but this area is very important to target. Excessive tightness in the calf muscles can negatively affect muscles higher up the leg and even into the lower back. If you engage in activities that involve jumping or being on your toes, like basketball, boxing, or jump rope, you could benefit from foam rolling the calf muscles. Even if you don't engage in activities like this, your calves are probably tight if you sit a lot or wear high heels!

Place the foam roller under your calf muscles, with your legs straight and your hands supporting most of your weight behind you or next to you, on either side of your hips. Lift your hips off the floor to place more pressure on your calves. Slowly roll along the roller, moving from the top of your ankle to just before the back of your knee. If you feel you need even more pressure on your muscles, lift one leg off the roller to roll one calf at a time, or stack one leg on top of the other. Roll with your feet turned in and out to massage the calves from different angles.

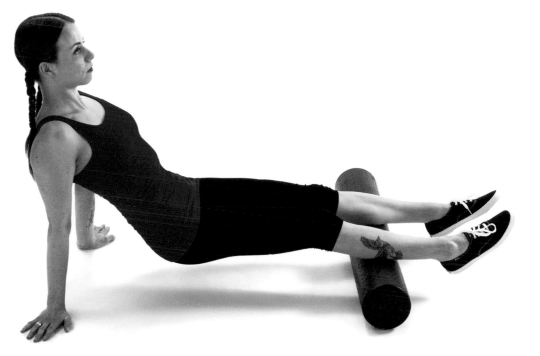

Piriformis

The piriformis is a small muscle located deep within the posterior pelvis, in the mid to upper buttock area. It is primarily responsible for rotating the leg outward from the hip. An excessively tight piriformis can cause sciatic pain in the buttock and down the leg by irritating the sciatic nerve. A tight piriformis muscle can also lead to limited range of motion in exercises such as squats and lunges.

Sit on the foam roller, with most of your weight on the right side of your glutes. Your piriformis is located near your hip joint in the upper/ mid buttock area; you'll most likely notice when you're on it, as in most people it's quite tight. If you'd like increased pressure on the piriformis, cross your right ankle over your left knee and roll over your piriformis in this position.

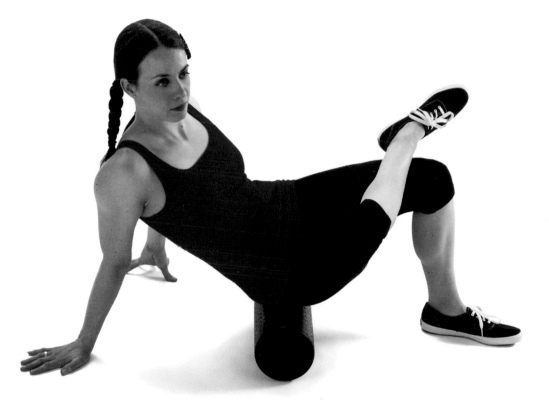

Glutes

The gluteus maximus is the largest muscle in the human body and is the most superficial (close to the surface) of all the gluteal muscles. The gluteus maximus covers the gluteus medius and the gluteus minimus, which are smaller muscles important to stabilizing the pelvis and assisting in leg movement at the hip. All these muscles can be rolled on the foam roller to release tension.

Place the foam roller under your glutes, with your hands on the floor behind you for support. Slowly roll across your glute muscles. You can also lean toward one side for more pressure on the muscle, rolling the lateral (outside) part of the muscle group as well. The gluteus maximus is the largest muscle in the body and can carry lots of tension, so make sure you spend time looking for trigger points and releasing tension from the glutes.

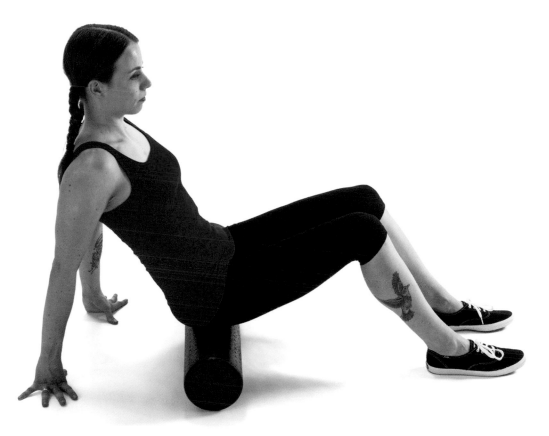

Latissimus dorsi

The latissimus dorsi muscles ("lats" for short) are the widest and most powerful muscles of the back. They create the sought-after V-shape in a well-conditioned person's upper back and torso. Foam rolling your lats may be especially beneficial after training them with exercises such as pull-ups, wide grip cable pull-downs, or dumbbell rows.

Lie on your right side with the foam roller placed under your right armpit. Extend your right arm along the floor. Slowly roll toward your waist, stopping just before you get to the bottom of your rib cage. Rotate your body slightly to the left to access the lats from a slightly different angle. Keep your left hand on the floor if this is feeling intense enough. If you need more pressure, remove your left hand from the floor.

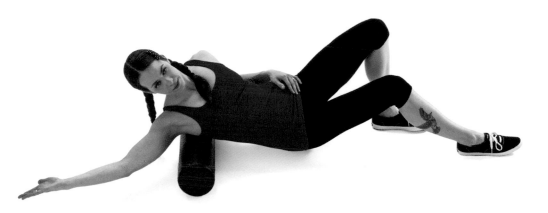

Upper back

The upper back is chronically tight in many, if not most, people. Every single client I've ever trained who has foam rolled his or her upper back has noticed at least some areas of tightness!

Position the foam roller lengthwise under your mid-back. Support your head with your hands, without pulling or pushing on your neck. Bend your knees and place your feet flat on the floor. Lift your hips off the floor. Roll slowly from your mid-back upward toward your head, stopping below the neck. Use your feet on the floor to control the motion and pressure, and tilt your body slightly from side to side to access the upper back muscles from different angles.

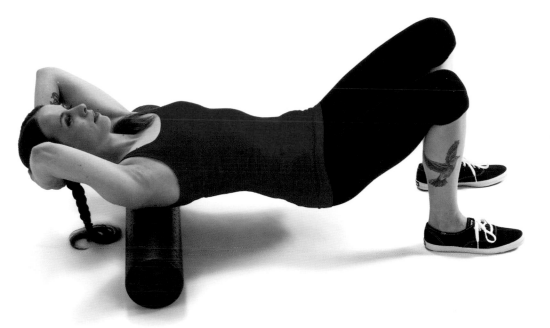

Upper back/rhomboids

Here's a variation of the previous upper back move, which targets the rhomboids. Your rhomboids squeeze your shoulder blades together.

Lie on the foam roller lengthwise, with your head at one end and your tailbone at the other end. Bend your knees and place your feet flat on the floor. With your elbows bent and hands near your head, carefully roll slightly from left to right, focusing on the muscles in your upper back and between your shoulder blades. Make sure you don't twist your spine as you roll; move your body as one unit. Try lifting your head slightly to access your upper back muscles from a different angle.

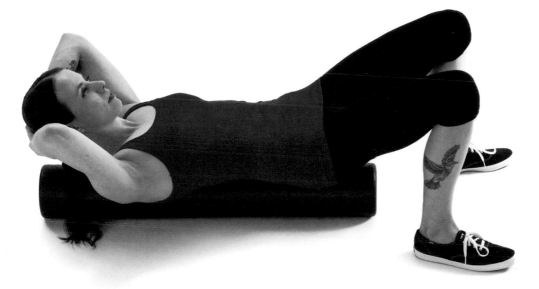

Anterior tibialis

The anterior tibialis is the most prominent shin muscle. It lies just laterally (to the outside of the body) of the shin along the front of your lower leg. The anterior tibialis serves to lift your toes off the ground with every step you take. It's often overlooked in foam rolling, but it's especially important for people who engage in activities such as running or rope jumping. If you've ever experienced shin splints, you know how painful this muscle can be when strained.

Start on your hands and knees, with the foam roller placed on your shins, just above your ankles. Tuck your knees toward your chest to roll along your shins, stopping just below the knee. Make sure you stay on the muscle, instead of putting pressure on the tibia bone. Change the angle by leaning to the left and then to the right for a few repetitions, so different areas of your shin muscle make contact with the roller.

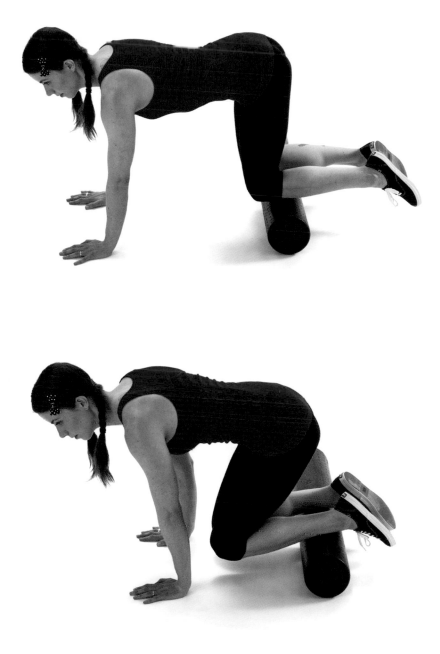

Peroneus

The peroneus can become very tight in athletes engaging in sports that include lots of lateral motion, like tennis; or jumping, like basketball. This muscle group is also often overused in runners, especially those who cover long distances.

Start on your right side, supporting your body on your right forearm, with the foam roller under the side of your calf muscle. Stack your left leg on top of your right, and rest your left arm on your side. Roll slowly from just above the ankle to just below the knee joint. If this is too intense and you need to back off on the pressure, place your left hand on the floor to support some of your weight.

Take care to stay on the fleshy part of your muscle, rather than putting pressure on the tibia bone.

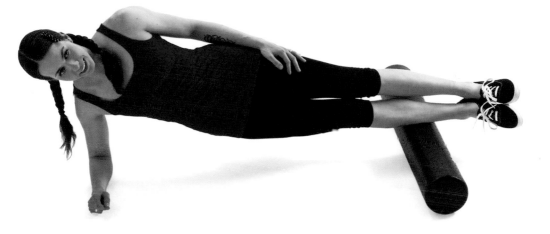

Adductors

The adductors are your inner thigh muscles. Foam rolling these muscles can be a bit awkward when it comes to positioning yourself on the roller, but don't neglect rolling this area just because it seems odd! Athletes in many different disciplines often encounter injuries to this muscle group, the most common of which is the groin strain or tear.

Option 1

Supporting yourself on your hands and knees, place the foam roller to the left of your left leg. With your knee bent, place your left inner thigh on the roller, keeping yourself supported by your hands (which should be placed directly under your shoulders). Your right leg is extended behind you on the floor. If this position doesn't provide enough pressure for you, lower down onto your forearms. Because of the somewhat awkward position your body is in, it's usually simplest to roll each half of the adductor muscle group separately. Start by rolling from just above the knee to halfway up your thigh. Complete slow repetitions, pausing on any sore spots, then reposition the roller and roll from mid-thigh to the groin.

Make sure you keep your core muscles braced throughout this movement, to prevent your lower back from sagging toward the floor.

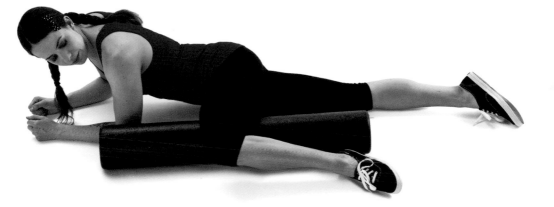

Option 2

This variation may be more challenging for people with limited flexibility, but because the hip isn't flexed in this position (compared to the flexed hip position in Option 1), it's easier to access the upper groin muscles that often hold the most tension. This includes the adductor brevis, the smallest and shortest of the adductor muscles.

Begin seated on the floor. Bend your right knee, resting your right thigh and lower leg on the floor. Extend your left leg and place the foam roller near the top of the left thigh. Place your hands on the floor for balance. You may need to rotate to the side somewhat to access the inner thigh muscles. Slowly roll back and forth along the inner thigh muscles of the left leg, then switch sides.

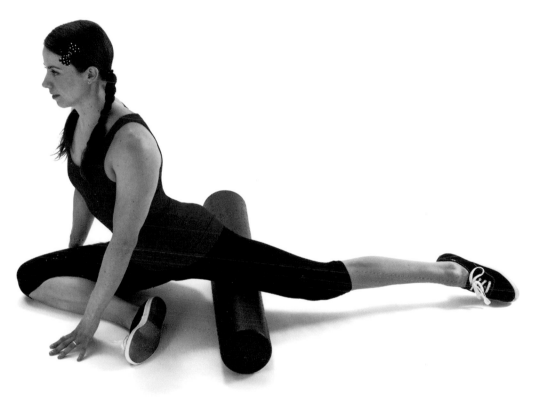

Tensor fasciae latae

The tensor fasciae latae–also known as the TFL–is a small muscle that originates in the upper anterior (front) portion of the pelvis, and attaches to the IT band. So the TFL runs from the top of the pelvis to the hip. The TFL can get strained in runners who increase their mileage too quickly, before the body has time to adjust. For people with IT band problems, rolling the TFL can be very effective. (Remember, rolling the IT band itself is a no-no.)

Assume a side-lying position with the foam roller placed under the upper thigh of the right leg. Ensure the roller is placed just below your pelvis. Rest your right forearm on the floor. Bend your left leg so your left foot rests on the floor in front of your extended right leg. You won't need to roll very far because this muscle is relatively small; a quarter of the way down your thigh will suffice.

Use both hands on the floor for less pressure on the TFL, or one hand on the floor for more pressure. Make sure you don't roll directly over your hip bone.

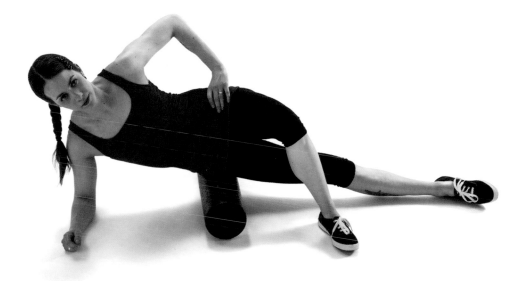

Triceps

Your triceps, located at the back of your arms, are major players in exercises such as push-ups and bench presses.

Lie on your right side with the foam roller placed under your right armpit. Extend your right arm along the floor. Slowly roll toward your elbow, stopping before you get to the elbow joint. Keep your left hand on the floor if this is feeling intense enough. If you need more pressure, remove your left hand from the floor.

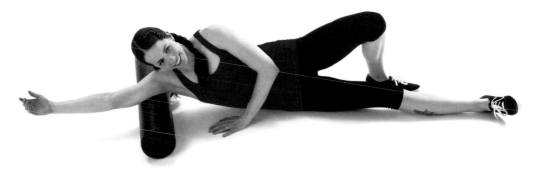

Pectorals

Pectoral (chest) muscles often become tight in people who have sedentary, seated jobs. Men can foam roll the entire width of their chests. For pretty obvious anatomical reasons, women will foam roll as much of the chest area as is comfortable.

Start lying prone on the floor with the foam roller placed parallel to your left side. Place your left arm on the roller, palm facing the floor. Move the roller so that it is placed on the inside of your armpit and shoulder. Slowly roll the roller toward the middle of your chest, stopping on any tender areas.

Try this massage move on a foam roller first. If you feel you need additional pressure or you find the position required for rolling your chest uncomfortable, try using a tennis ball, baseball, or lacrosse ball instead. You can also try this standing against a wall, with the ball wedged between the wall and your chest muscle.

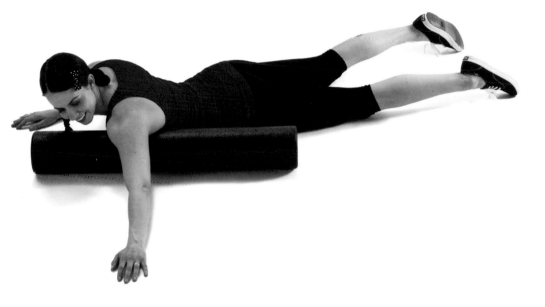

Neck

The neck muscles supporting the head are very common tight spots. From people who sit in front of a computer screen all day to competitive athletes, tightness in these muscles often causes tension headaches. When using a foam roller to release these muscles, there's no need to apply extra pressure. It may actually be dangerous to your neck and head, also known as the cervical spine area. Just relax and let the weight of your head release your neck muscles.

Lie on the ground with your knees bent and feet flat on the floor. With the foam roller perpendicular to your body, place your neck on the foam roller and relax your neck muscles so your head is supported by the roller. You can slowly move your head from side to side, holding for 30 seconds or more when you find tender areas.

Don't add any additional pressure to your neck area when performing this move. The weight of your head is enough!

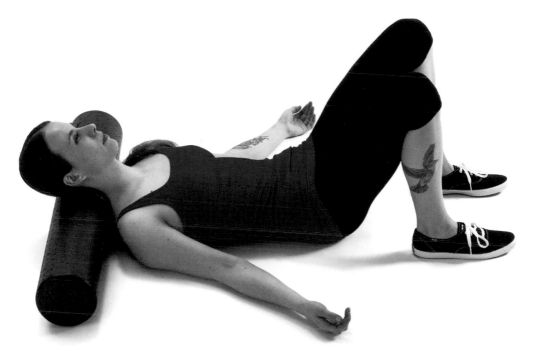

Biceps

Tight biceps muscles can sometimes lead to forearm pain, especially if you lift weights regularly. Foam rolling your biceps may be especially useful after weight lifting movements targeting your back (biceps are an assistant muscle in these exercises), and of course movements targeting the biceps themselves (any curling movements, like barbell curls, dumbbell curls, or cable curls).

Lie on the floor on your right side. Extend your right arm and place your biceps muscle on the foam roller, using your left hand on the floor for stability. Roll from just below the shoulder to just above the elbow, staying on the fleshy part of the biceps muscle.

You can also try placing the foam roller on a kitchen table or massage table and bending down to roll your biceps, so you don't have to lie on the floor.

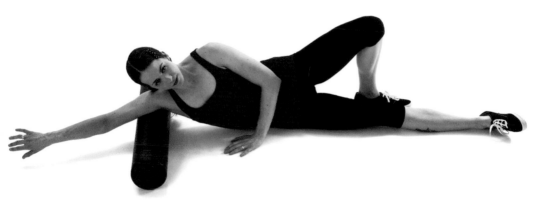

Forearms

Tight forearm muscles are more common than you may think. People with office jobs who spend long hours at a computer are at risk for developing tight forearm muscles and overuse injuries such as repetitive strain syndrome or tendonitis. Many athletes and others who are regularly active can also develop tight forearm muscles, like tennis players and weight lifters, for instance.

This move is most easily completed with the roller placed on a table. Stand in front of a table (e.g. a massage table or a kitchen table), with the roller placed crosswise in front of you. Extend your arms in front of you with your palms facing up. Place your forearms on the roller, and slowly move back and forth to roll your forearms from just above the wrist to just below the elbow.

If you don't have a table available (say, at the gym after a weight lifting session), you can kneel on the floor in front of the roller. Extend your arms, place them on the roller with your palms facing up, and lean forward and backward to roll along your forearms.

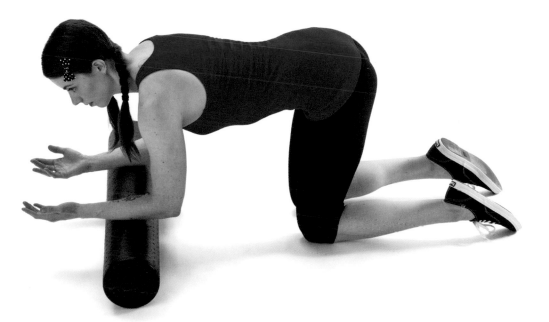

STRENGTH & CORE STABILITY

You can get a great core stability and balance workout using a half roller or a full roller for any exercise, whether or not it's focused on the core. In most of the core-specific exercises, you can vary the difficulty of your workout by the type of foam roller you use. For exercises like roll-outs, you need to use a full foam roller as the half ones don't roll along the floor. Most other core exercises, though, have a few difficulty level options. If you're just starting out, use a half roller with the curved side up and flat side down. Progress from there by flipping it the other way around, so you have the flat side up and the curved side down. If you're really up for a challenge, use a full foam roller.

Other exercises in the Strength and Core Stability section don't focus on the core muscles in particular, but work them nonetheless. For example, performing a push-up with your hands on a foam roller is most challenging for the upper body muscles, but your core muscles are challenged at the same time because you need to keep your balance on the roller.

Dead bug

Lie lengthwise on a half foam roller, with your head at one end and your tailbone at the other. Make sure your back is flat against the roller; engage your core muscles to ensure you maintain this position throughout the exercise. Extend your arms toward the ceiling, keeping them straight. Flex your hips and knees to bring your thighs perpendicular to the floor, and your lower legs parallel to the floor. This is the starting position (which requires a great deal of balance).

Keeping your abs tight so your lower back doesn't arch, extend your right arm above your head while extending your left leg toward the floor. Hold for a count, then return to the start position and repeat on the other side.

Make sure the entire length of your back stays in contact with the foam roller at all times. Also make sure you're extending each leg fully, bringing it as close to the ground as possible without actually making contact with the floor.

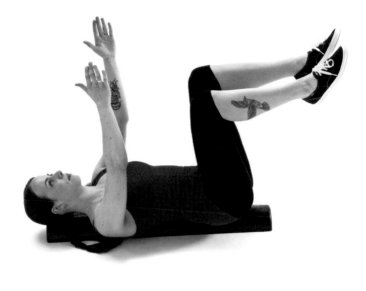

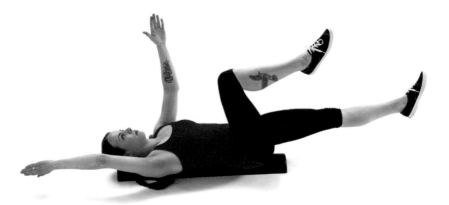

Roll-outs

Ready for a challenging core exercise? This move targets your anterior (front) and posterior (back) core muscles to provide stability as you complete the exercise.

Kneel with the foam roller in front of you. Use a yoga or exercise mat under your knees if you like. Place your forearms on the foam roller, shoulder width apart. Tighten your abdominal muscles by drawing your belly button toward your spine. Slowly roll the foam roller, one arm at a time, away from your body. Your body will begin to form a straight line from your knees to your head, and your arms will stretch out in front of you. Pause at the extended position, then slowly roll your way back to the starting position.

The farther away from your body you roll, the more challenging this exercise will feel. It's very important to go only so far as your core strength can handle. Make sure you don't roll so far that your lower back sags toward the floor.

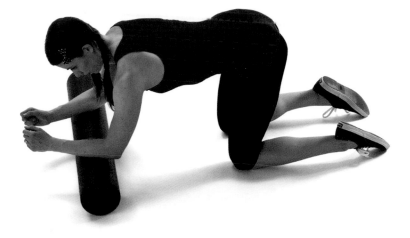

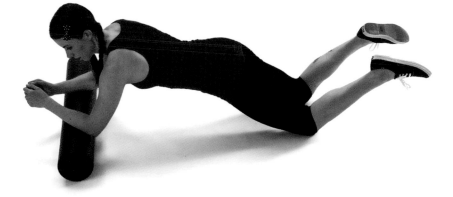

Leg extensions

Leg extensions focus on the lower abdominal muscles, since they need to stabilize your pelvis as you move your leg, and keep you balanced on the foam roller at the same time.

Lie lengthwise on the foam roller with your head at one end and your tailbone at the other. Bend your legs so your feet are on the floor, about hip width apart. Ensure your entire back is flat against the foam roller, and tighten your abdominal muscles by drawing your belly button toward your spine. Rest your arms on your chest; the challenge of this move comes from not using your arms for balance. Keeping your abdominals very tight, slowly extend your left leg until it is straight. Hold for a few counts, then return your left foot to the ground and repeat on the right.

The closer together you bring your feet, the less stable (and thus, the more challenging) this move becomes. Make sure that no part of your back loses contact with the foam roller throughout this exercise.

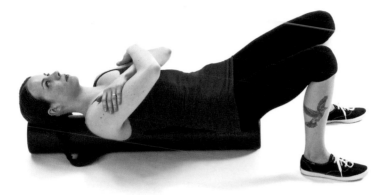

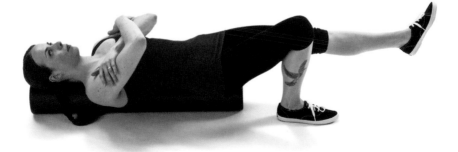

Weighted overhead reaches

Using weight is a great way to challenge your abs while on the foam roller. You can use anything you like for added weight, including medicine balls, dumbbells, or household objects like large books or full beverage containers if you're at home with no exercise equipment.

Lie lengthwise on the foam roller with your head at one end and your tailbone at the other. Bend your legs so your feet are on the floor, about hip width apart. Ensure your entire back is flat against the foam roller, and tighten your abdominal muscles by drawing your belly button toward your spine. Hold a weighted object in both hands and extend your arms straight up toward the ceiling. Keeping your abs engaged and your arms straight, slowly reach your arms overhead. Pause, then slowly return to the arms straight up (perpendicular to the floor) position and repeat.

The closer together you bring your feet, the less stable (and thus, the more challenging) this move becomes. Increasing the weight you use for this exercise also increases its difficulty. Make sure that no part of your back loses contact with the foam roller throughout this exercise.

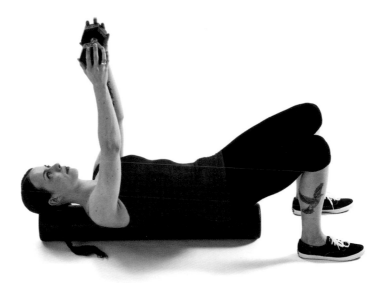

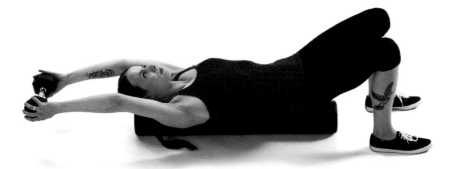

Weighted side-to-side reaches

Here's a variation of the basic overhead weighted reach that focuses more on your oblique abdominal muscles.

Lie lengthwise on the foam roller with your head at one end and your tailbone at the other. Bend your legs so your feet are on the floor, about hip width apart. Ensure your entire back is flat against the foam roller, and tighten your abdominal muscles by drawing your belly button toward your spine. Hold a weighted object in both hands and extend your arms straight up toward the ceiling. Keeping your abs engaged and your arms straight, slowly reach your arms to one side. Pause, then slowly return to the arms straight up (perpendicular to the floor) position and repeat by reaching to the other side.

Make sure you keep your body in alignment as you reach to the side. The closer together you bring your feet, the less stable (and thus, the more challenging) this move becomes. Increasing the weight you use for this exercise also increases its difficulty. Make sure that no part of your back loses contact with the foam roller throughout this exercise.

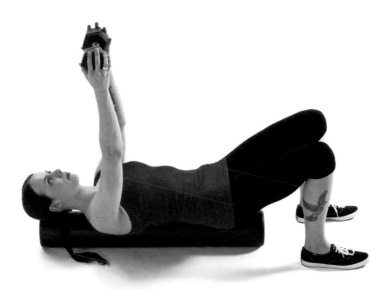

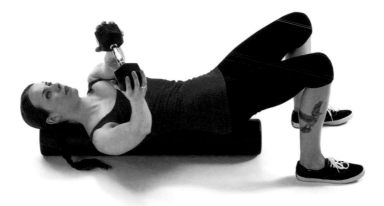

Alternate leg lowering

Once you're comfortable performing leg extensions, try this leg lowering exercise for more of a core challenge.

Lie lengthwise on the foam roller with your head at one end and your tailbone at the other. Bend your legs so your feet are on the floor, about hip width apart. Ensure your entire back is flat against the foam roller, and tighten your abdominal muscles by drawing your belly button toward your spine. Using your arms as lightly as possible on the floor for balance, bring both legs straight toward the ceiling. Keeping your back completely flat against the roller, slowly straighten your right leg, bringing your heel toward the floor (but don't actually touch the floor). Pause, then slowly bring your right leg back to the start position and repeat with your left leg.

If you feel any part of your back losing contact with the foam roller as you lower your leg, stop and return to the start position even if you haven't brought your heel very close to the ground. As you increase your core strength, you'll be able to reach your leg farther toward the ground without arching your back.

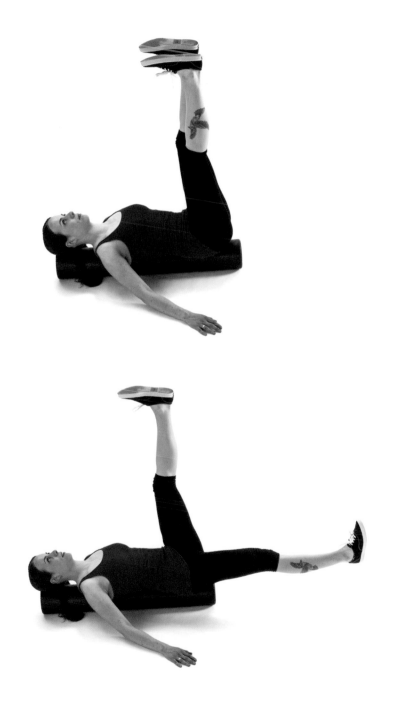

Bicycle crunches

Bicycle crunches are a great way to engage a large portion of the abdominal muscles, including the lower abdominals, transverse abdominus, and obliques.

Lie lengthwise on the foam roller with your head at one end and your tailbone at the other. Bend your legs so your feet are on the floor, about hip width apart. Bend your arms and lightly touch the back of your head without interlacing your fingers. Contract your abs and raise your upper back off the foam roller. Lift your right leg off the floor as you twist your torso, aiming your left pectoral muscle toward your right knee. Lower to the start position and repeat, aiming your right pectoral toward your left knee.

Make sure you don't use your hands to pull on your head or neck. Initiate the movement from your abdominals, and keep your elbows wide out to the sides.

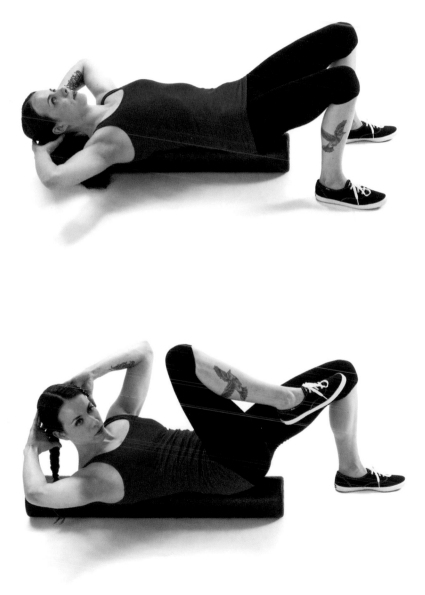

Tucks

This exercise is often performed using a stability ball. It engages the entire core, with a focus on the lower abdominals.

Start in a plank position, with your hands directly under your shoulders and your entire body in a straight line. The foam roller is placed on your shins, just under your knees. Tighten your abdominal muscles by drawing your belly button toward your spine. Now tuck your knees toward your chest, keeping your core muscles contracted. The foam roller will roll along your lower legs, toward your feet. Pause in the contracted position, then extend your legs back into the plank position.

Make sure your lower back doesn't "sag" toward the floor as you bring your legs back to the starting position after the tuck.

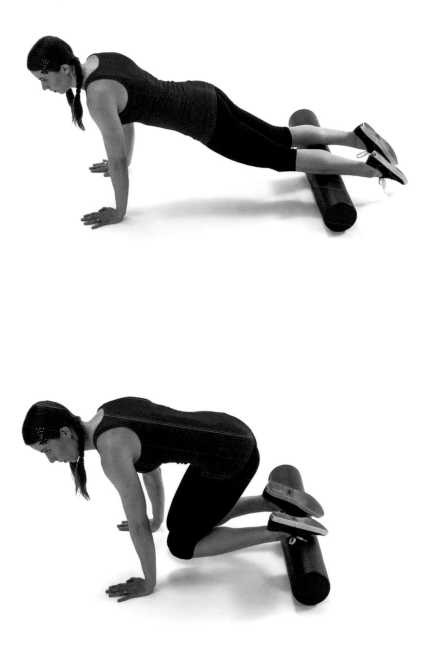

Reverse tucks

This move works your core as well as your posterior chain (lower back, glutes, and hamstrings).

Start in a seated position with your ankles on the foam roller and your hands beside your hips. Keep your arms and legs straight as you lift your hips off the floor. Extend your legs into a reverse plank position, forming a straight line from your chest to your feet. The roller will roll up your calves. Hold briefly, then use your abdominal muscles to pull your hips back underneath and behind you as far as you can. Hold this position, then return to the plank position.

Make sure you keep your chest up throughout the movement, and try to prevent your back from rounding in the tucked position.

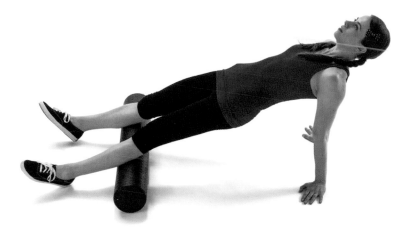

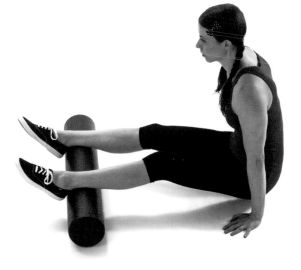

Reverse lunge

This move strengthens the muscles of your lower body, while also challenging your balance. As a bonus, you'll get tension release foam rolling along each shin as you complete this exercise.

Start in a standing position with the foam roller placed behind you, hands on your hips. Place your right foot on top of the foam roller. Now extend your right leg behind you as you bend your left knee into a lunge position. The roller will roll along your right shin toward your knee. When your left knee is at a 90-degree angle (your thigh is parallel to the floor), pause, then return to the start position.

Remember to maintain perfect posture throughout this exercise, keeping your shoulder blades squeezed and your back straight.

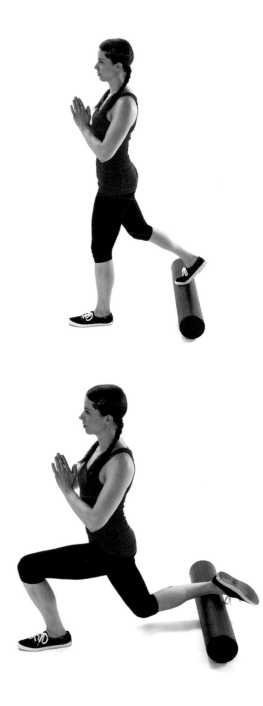

Reverse crunch

Holding a foam roller between the backs of your ankles and thighs prevents you from using any momentum in this exercise. This ensures you're working the intended muscles: your abdominals!

Lie on your back with a foam roller wedged between the backs of your ankles and thighs. Maintain this position with the foam roller throughout the exercise. Place your arms on the floor alongside your body. Tighten your abdominal muscles by drawing your belly button toward your spine. Lift your hips off the floor, bringing your knees toward your chest as far as you can go. Slowly return to the start position and repeat for reps.

If you want to try a more challenging variation of this move, bring your arms overhead and hold on to a heavy object (like a dumbbell or medicine ball) while performing this exercise. If you're looking for the most difficult variation possible, perform this move with arms overhead, not holding on to any counterweight.

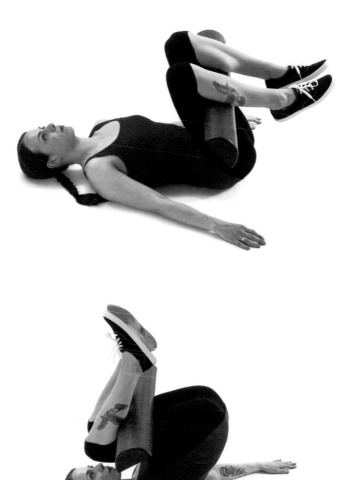

Push-up

Here's a push-up variation that works your core more than standard push-ups. If you're not able to do full push-ups from your toes, try this move resting on your knees instead.

Start in a plank position with your toes on the floor and your hands placed on the foam roller, directly underneath your shoulders. Contract your abdominal muscles. Lower yourself into a push-up position by bending your arms and bringing your chest as close to the foam roller as possible. Push up using your chest and triceps muscles to return to the starting position and repeat for reps.

Make sure that your body stays in one straight line, without sagging your lower back toward the floor or craning your neck forward. Keep the foam roller as stable as possible throughout the movement. For a variation, try this exercise with your feet placed on the roller and your hands on the floor. The closer together you bring your feet on the roller, the more challenging the move will become.

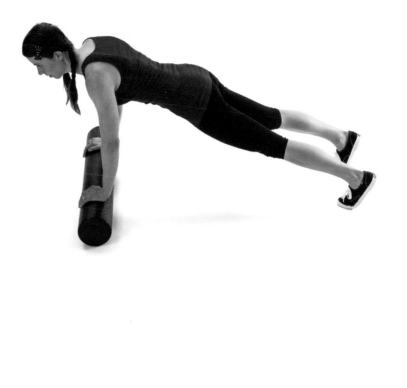

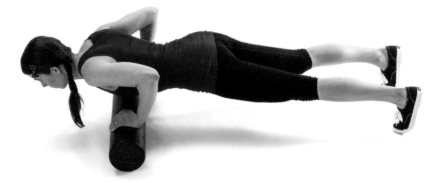

Glute bridge

The glute bridge is a classic glute, hamstring, and lower back strengthener. The foam roller makes this exercise more challenging than performing it with your feet on the ground.

Option 1: Both feet on the roller

Lie supine on the floor, with your knees bent and your feet placed hip width apart on the foam roller close to your glutes. Your arms should be resting at your sides, palms facing down. Tighten your core muscles and press through your feet to lift your body off the floor. Most of your weight will be supported by your upper back and feet, and your body should form a straight line from your upper back to your knees. Squeeze your glutes in this position. You can hold this position as a static (isometric) exercise, or perform slow repetitions by returning to the start position and repeating the exercise.

The farther away from your glutes you position the foam roller, the more challenging this move will become (and the more your hamstring muscles will work).

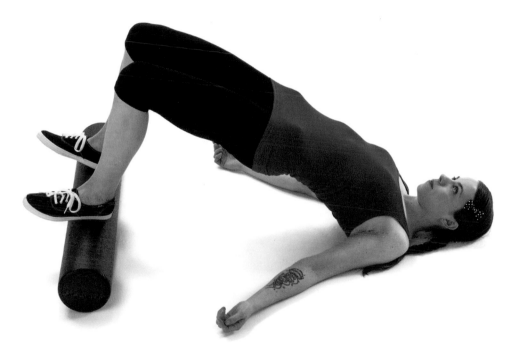

Option 2: One-legged glute bridge

This is a more challenging version of the regular glute bridge, working your glutes, hamstrings, and lower back.

Lie supine on the floor, with your knees bent and your feet placed hip width apart on the foam roller close to your glutes. Your arms should be resting at your sides, palms facing down. Lift your left foot off the roller, straightening your leg. Now tighten your core muscles and press through your right foot to lift your body off the floor. Most of your weight will be supported by your upper back and right leg, and your body should form a straight line from your upper back to your right knee. You can hold this position as a static (isometric) exercise, or perform slow repetitions by returning to the start position and repeating the exercise. Once you've completed the exercise with your right foot on the roller, switch sides so your left leg is on the roller and your right leg is straight in the air.

The farther away from your glutes you position the foam roller, the more challenging this move will become (and the more your hamstring muscles will work).

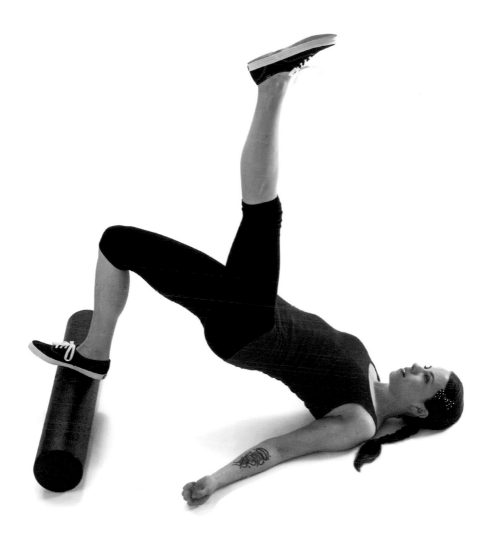

High plank with leg lifts

This exercise challenges your core to stabilize your body as you lift your legs.

Option 1: Hands on roller

Start in a high plank position with your hands shoulder width apart on the foam roller and your toes on the floor. Make sure your head is in line with your spine and that you maintain a rigid position from shoulders to ankles. Brace your abdominal muscles to prevent your lower back from "sagging" toward the floor. Slowly lift your right leg off the floor, hold for a second or two, and then return your foot to the floor. Repeat with your left leg.

Try to keep the roller as stable as possible throughout the movement.

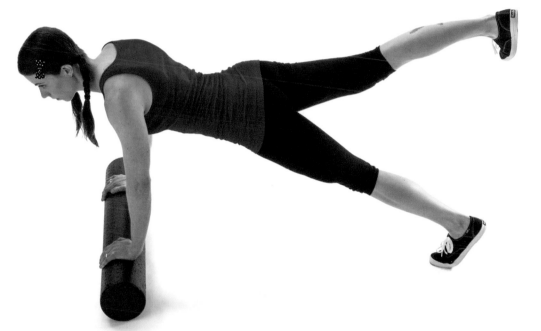

Option 2: Feet on roller

Start in a high plank position with your hands under your shoulders and toes on the foam roller. Make sure your head is in line with your spine and that you maintain a rigid position from shoulders to ankles. Prevent your lower back from "sagging" toward the floor by bracing your abdominal muscles. Slowly lift your right leg off the roller, hold for a second or two, and then return your foot to the roller. Repeat with your left leg.

Try to keep the roller as stable as possible throughout the movement.

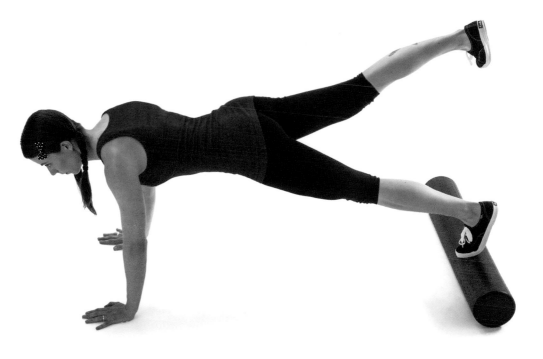

V-sit with alternating arm raises

This exercise challenges your abdominal muscles to hold a static (isometric) position with only a small point of stabilization (your hand on the floor).

Sit in the middle of the foam roller with your feet on the ground to either side. Using your hands on the floor for balance, bring both legs to a table-top position, contracting your abdominal muscles and keeping your chest up and shoulders back. Now reach your left arm up toward the ceiling. Try to use as little of your right hand on the floor as possible for balance. Try using just your fingers! Now slowly switch arms so your left fingers are lightly placed on the floor, and your right arm reaches toward the ceiling.

Try to keep your chest as "proud" as possible throughout this movement, in an effort to prevent your back from rounding.

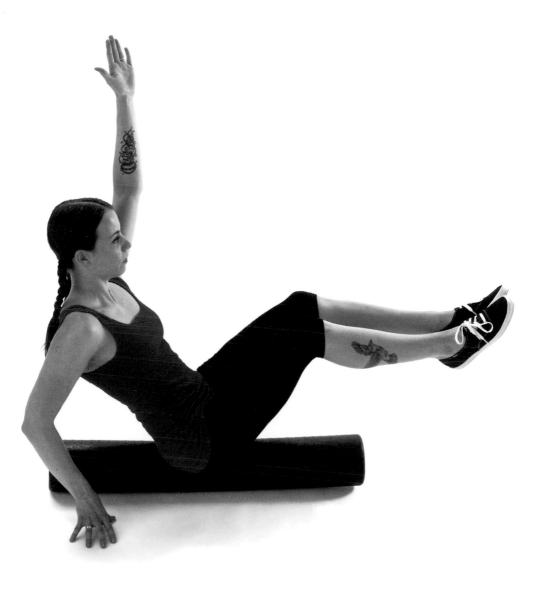

Mountain climber

This exercise adds instability to the standard mountain climber exercise, which means it's more challenging for your core muscles. Regular mountain climbers (same exercise but without the foam roller) are performed quickly, jumping each leg in and out. This is a conditioning exercise that involves strength and also cardio capacity. Foam roller mountain climbers are performed more slowly, focusing on maintaining balance and contracting the abdominal muscles.

Begin in a plank position with your toes on the floor and your hands placed on the foam roller, directly underneath your shoulders. Contract your abdominal muscles. Flex your right hip and knee to tuck your knee toward your chest. Pause briefly, contracting your abdominal muscles as much as you can, then return to the start position and repeat on the left side.

For a greater challenge, perform this exercise with your hands flat on the floor, and your feet on the foam roller, about hip width apart (toes are resting on the foam roller). Try to keep the roller as stable as possible throughout both variations of the movement.

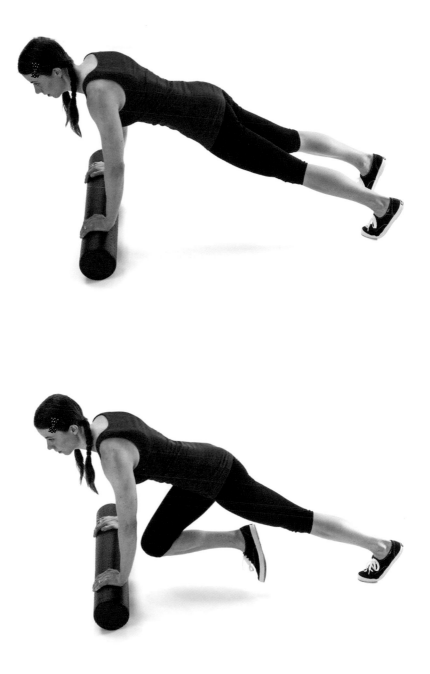

Split squat

Challenge your balance and stability by performing this classic lower body move on a half foam roller instead of on the floor.

Stand on a half foam roller with hands on your hips or clasped in front of your chest, left foot forward and right foot back. Squat down by flexing your left knee and hip. Your left knee should form a 90-degree angle, and your right knee should almost touch the roller. Straighten both legs to return to the start position, complete reps, then switch sides.

Make sure you maintain perfect posture throughout this exercise, keeping your shoulder blades squeezed together and your back straight. For a more challenging variation, perform this move on a half roller with the flat side facing up.

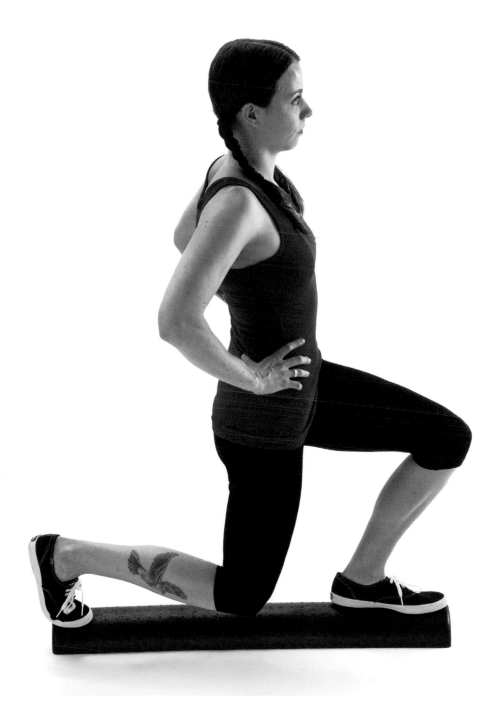

Squat

With three options for difficulty level, this move will really challenge your balance. It reminds me of surfing!

Start with a half foam roller flat side down on the floor. Step onto the roller with both feet. Your feet should be hip width apart, or a little wider. Stand tall with good posture, then bend at the hips and knees, sending your hips and your glutes behind you to perform a squat. Use your arms outstretched in front of you for balance, if needed, or clasp your hands together in front of your chest (more difficult). Return to the start position and repeat the movement.

For a more advanced version, flip over the half foam roller and complete this exercise with the flat side up. If you're really up for a balance challenge, do this exercise on a full, circular foam roller. Be careful and make sure you have a chair or other support object nearby in case you need it.

Keep your back straight throughout the movement, and your head in line with your spine.

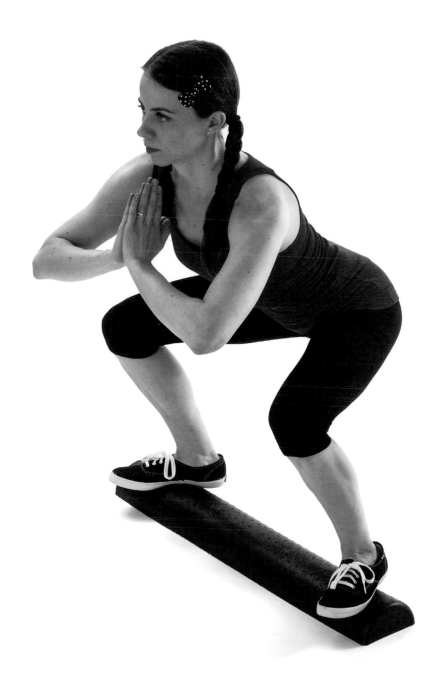

Bird-dog

The bird-dog is a classic core stability move performed in personal training studios everywhere. This one incorporates a foam roller for a fresh twist on an old classic.

Start on all fours with your hands placed directly under your shoulders, and your shins placed onto the foam roller. Your knees should be directly under your hips. Tighten your abdominal muscles as you raise your right arm, bringing it parallel to the floor. At the same time, lift your left leg off the roller and extend it behind you, squeezing your left glute at the top of the motion. Pause briefly, then return to the start position and repeat on the other side.

Ensure you keep both your arm and leg straight as you lift them. Also make sure you keep the roller as still as possible, and your hips square with your shoulders.

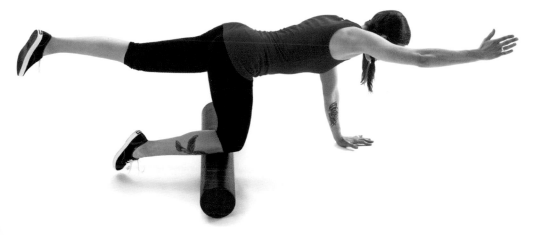

Side plank with leg lift

Adding a foam roller to this classic exercise adds a level of instability, making this move more challenging for your core muscles.

With the foam roller placed under the outside of your left leg, support yourself on your left forearm. Your left elbow should be placed directly under your left shoulder. Press through your left forearm and left leg, lifting your hips off the ground to create a straight line from your head to your feet. Make sure you keep your hips stacked, with no tilting forward or backward. Once you feel stable in this position, lift your right leg and hold.

Ensure that your body doesn't sag toward the floor. Keep your abdominal muscles tight throughout the exercise. If you're up for a greater challenge, try this exercise with just your hand supporting your weight on the ground, instead of your forearm. In this variation your entire arm will be straight, with your hand directly under your shoulder.

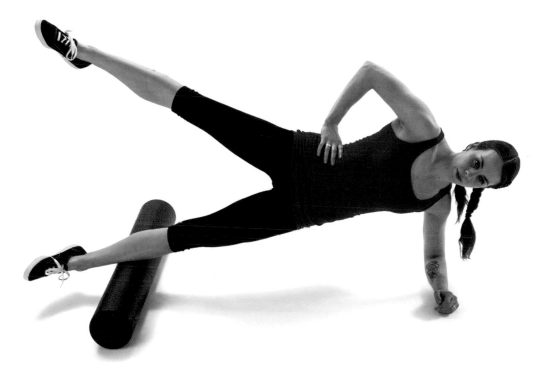

Reverse plank with leg lift

Challenge your upper body strength and your isometric (static hold) hamstring strength with this exercise.

Start in a seated position, with your legs straight, ankles on the foam roller, and hands under your shoulders with fingers facing forwards or to the side. Keeping your arms straight, lift your hips off the floor and bring your body into a reverse plank, creating a straight line from your chest to your feet. Squeeze your glutes to keep your hips in line with the rest of your body, and squeeze your shoulder blades together. Now lift your right leg off the roller, hold for a count, then return it to the roller and repeat on the left side. Once reps are completed, lower your hips back down to the floor to finish the exercise.

Make sure you keep both legs straight throughout this movement. Also ensure that your body stays in a straight line from your head to your supporting leg on the roller as you lift your opposite leg.

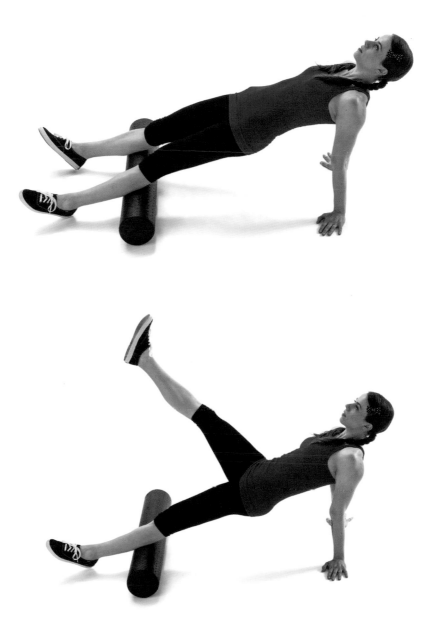

Obstacle course

This is your chance to get creative! Challenge your dynamic balance by setting up your own obstacle course made of foam rollers.

Set up several foam rollers of different sizes, shapes, and densities, then carefully walk along them, stepping over obstacles and keeping your balance. If you're using half foam rollers, place some with the rounded side up, and others with the flat side up. You can even try walking along the foam rollers sideways.

If you're up for an extra challenge, try placing objects along the course for you to pick up, while balancing on a foam roller.

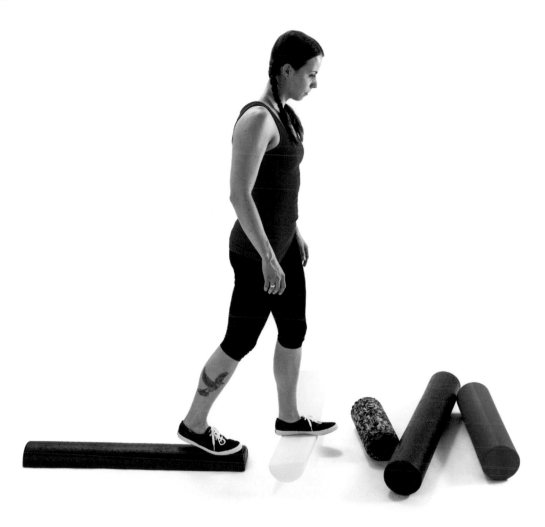

Acknowledgments

I'd like to thank all the remarkable people who helped and supported me while working on this project. Most importantly, I thank Abigail Gehring and her team at Skyhorse Publishing for the opportunity to write this book.

My thanks to John Watson of Image Maker Photographic Studio for his excellent photography and hard work during our full day of shooting for this book.

I would like to acknowledge the contributions of the five health and fitness professionals who shared their expertise: Angela Kromidas, Faolan Dunphy, Gemma Doyle, Karen Martens, and Naomi Canales. Their knowledge deepened the scope of information I could present to readers.

Big thanks to all my amazing clients, many of whom were guinea pigs for the foam roller exercises in this book, especially Allison, Annaliese, Carmen, Cheri, Elke, Fiona, Ian, Isabelle, Jenny, Jonathan, Kensi, Nicole, Peter, Ron, Sally, Sarita, Sylvia, Tania, Tony, and Waylin: you continue to make my work not seem like work.

I'd like to thank my editing team Doris Jetz, Jonathan Wong, Meika Kiven, and Nicole Pointon. They provided insightful feedback and editing of the final book manuscript within a very tight deadline. You guys are awesome!

An extra special shout-out to my best friend Setareh Bateni and my "G's": Heidi Braacx, Kevin Lee, and Holly Burton. Thanks for always rooting for me, and for your lifelong friendships. And to my bright, patient, kind, and incredibly good-looking husband Murray: thank you for your continued support of all my crazy projects, keeping me sane and reminding me to take breaks, your insight into my work, and your delicious dinners.

INDEX